Your Heart Needs the
Mediterranean Diet

Your Heart Needs the Mediterranean Diet

Learn How Mediterraneans Have Kept a Healthy Heart for Centuries

Emilia Klapp, R.D, B.S.

PREVENTIVE NUTRITION PRESS
SOUTH PASADENA, CALIFORNIA

First printing 2007

ISBN 978-0-9791260-3-1
LCCN 2007920427

ATTENTION CORPORATIONS, UNIVERSITIES, COLLEGES, AND PROFESSIONAL ORGANIZATIONS: Quantity discounts are available on bulk purchases of this book for educational, gift purposes, or as premiums for increasing magazine subscriptions or renewals. Special books or book excerpts can also be created to fit specific needs. For information, please contact Preventive Nutrition Press, P.O. Box 1227, South Pasadena, CA 91031; (626) 441-4780.

To my daughter Nadia

Table of Contents

Why Did I Write This Book? . . . . *ix*

Chapter One
What Is the Mediterranean Diet? *1*

Chapter Two
Physical Activity: A Magical Pill *13*

Chapter Three
The Sinister Connection:
High Blood Pressure and Processed Foods *23*

Chapter Four
Fruits and Vegetables:
Your Heart's Friends *35*

Chapter Five
Fruits and Vegetables:
Medicine of the Future *47*

Chapter Six
Tomatoes: A Staple Food for Your Heart *59*

Chapter Seven
Is Fat the Villain? *67*

Chapter Eight
If It Has a Mother and a Father,
It Has Cholesterol *83*

Chapter Nine
Olive Oil: "Liquid Gold" *97*

Chapter Ten
Legumes and Whole Grains:
The Cholesterol-Fiber Link *109*

Chapter Eleven
Garlic Can Protect Us
From More Than Vampires *123*

Glossary *137*

Index *143*

Why Did I Write This Book?

In the early 1990s, my mother and three of my best friends passed away at very young ages. Crushed and bewildered by these unexpected losses, I became a voracious reader of anything published in the area of nutrition in an attempt to understand what had happened and whether these untimely deaths could have been prevented. As I read, it became clear to me that modern medicine does not have all the answers. Unless we take control of our bodies and practice prevention, we might not reach old age. Or even if we do, we might not enjoy the best possible health.

What I read also became a wake-up call for me. I realized that not only was I ignoring many of the healthy habits I grew up with in Spain, my country of origin, but my diet could be described as "reckless." I ate few fruits and vegetables; my intake of saturated fat was way over the limit; and I was on the verge of becoming a sugar addict (on my trips to the supermarket my first stop was invariably the cookie and candy aisles). Basically, if I were to continue with this diet, eventually I would have wound up in the place I feared most: the doctor's office.

As I began to realize that the secret to good health lies in how we nourish our bodies as well as in adequate physical activity, I felt compelled to spread the word. I was so excited about my findings I became a full-time pest to friends and family, constantly lecturing them on what to eat or what not to eat. It didn't take long to realize that for people to listen to what I had to say, I would need to have a formal education. So I went back to college and became a Registered Dietitian. And now, the same way I felt driven to tell family and friends how to prevent disease, I would like to share with you, through this book, what nutrition science has proven to be a good course of action.

This book also has a second goal: to help you realize that a healthy lifestyle does not have to mean deprivation or sacrifices. Is it really possible to enjoy a delicious meal that is also healthy? Of course! People in the Mediterranean countries do it all the time, and they are notorious for being among the healthiest people on earth. Because the Mediterranean diet has worked for its people for centuries in warding off many of the chronic diseases that plague us now, such as heart disease, stroke, diabetes, and obesity, why not copy it? And that's exactly what we are going to do.

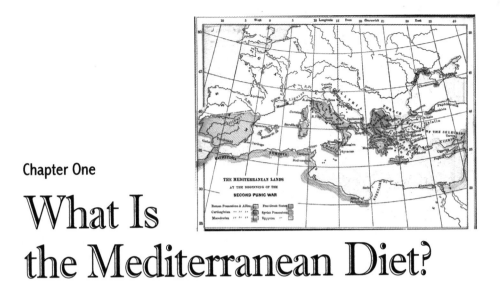

Chapter One

What Is the Mediterranean Diet?

Counseling Session—Day 1
Monday, 4:00 P.M.

Characters: Al, Patient; Emi, Registered Dietitian
Setting: Los Angeles, California. Emi is in her office waiting for her client, Al, who has been diagnosed with high blood pressure as well as high levels of cholesterol and triglycerides. Al is 43 years old, 5 feet 11 inches, and weighs 174 pounds. He works as a quality control manager in the airline industry. He is married and has two children in middle school. At 4:00 P.M. Al enters the room.

Introduction

Emi (*Shaking hands*): Good afternoon, Al. I'm delighted to finally meet you. Did you have any problem finding my office?

Al: Not at all. I just followed your directions.

Emi: Great! Have a seat, please. Would you like something to drink—water, tea?

Al: Water, please.

Emi (*Placing a glass of water on the table next to Al*): When we talked on the phone you told me that your last physical exam showed high levels of *cholesterol* and *triglycerides* as well as *high blood pressure*. Is that correct?

1

Al (*Looking worried*): Yes, although I am not sure what triglycerides means.

Emi: I know the word sounds showy but "triglycerides" is just the scientific name for *fat*, the fat you see in food and in the body. So, when you hear the word triglycerides, think fat.

Al: Is that all? It sure sounds intimidating! Anyhow, when my doctor saw my test results, he immediately wrote me a prescription to see you. According to him, I need to make a few changes in my lifestyle to reverse these health conditions. Otherwise, he said, I am headed for a *heart attack* or a *stroke*. He really scared me! So, here I am.

Emi: Did you bring the lab slip with your test results?

Al: Yes. (*Pulling the slip from his wallet*) Here.

TABLE #1—AL'S LAB RESULTS

Total Cholesterol	240 mg/dl (milligrams per deciliter)
LDL Cholesterol	150 mg/dl
HDL Cholesterol	42 mg/dl
Triglycerides	180 mg/dl
High blood pressure	160/80 mm HG (millimeters of mercury)

Emi: Thank you. You mentioned on the phone that you have a lot of stress in your life. Anything in particular that is causing it?

Al: Yes, my job! There are always deadlines to be met, employees who don't show up to work—I could go on and on. In addition, because of high gas prices and terrorist threats, I fear people may stop flying. If we don't need airplanes anymore, I'll lose my job!

Emi: Well, the global economy is causing more and more people to fly, so I wouldn't worry about that happening anytime soon.

Al: And then, there are my two children! Sometimes my wife works evenings, and I have to cook for everyone. I don't mind doing it, but no matter what I make, they always complain. That's why many times I resort to frozen dinners.

Emi: I understand what you are going through, but I am confident that little by little we'll be able to change a few things around —including how your children feel about your cooking.

Al: I hope so.

Emi: Well, let me say first that I am happy you came. And your doctor is right; high blood pressure and high levels of fat in the blood—cholesterol and triglycerides—can be reversed in many instances with the right nutrition and regular physical activity. On the other hand, if you don't change the behavior that has triggered these conditions, things will get worse and you may end up with a major health problem on your hands. I don't want to scare you, but your test results are not good. Are you ready and willing to take the necessary steps to correct your health condition?

Al: Yes, because I don't want to end up like my friend John, who has a lot of heart problems. What I don't understand is what has caused my lab values to be high, because I follow a very normal diet.

Emi: Probably a combination of things, such as lack of physical activity, eating too much of the wrong foods, too little of the right ones, and being subjected to a lot of stress. We'll find out. In the meantime, based on your doctor's prescription, we'll schedule eight counseling sessions where the two of us will work together to explore lifestyle changes that will help you correct and maintain normal levels of fat in the blood as well as a healthy blood pressure. To achieve this goal, our discussions will center on the *Mediterranean diet.*

Al: That sounds familiar. What kind of diet is that?

What Is the Mediterranean Diet?

Emi: The term "Mediterranean diet" refers to nutritional patterns found in countries along the Mediterranean basin where lifestyle has historically been associated with good health. Life expectancy in these countries is among the highest in the world, and heart disease and other diet-related diseases among the lowest. Scientists all over the world are now taking a second look at the effects the Mediterranean diet has on people's health. Two major studies conducted in Europe, EPIC and PREDIMED, showed that people who followed a Mediterranean diet based on fruits, vegetables, grains, and healthy fats aged at a lower rate and lived longer. These studies have also shown that this diet can lower blood pressure and cholesterol.[1]

Al: That's great!

Emi: Yes. Actually, we can say that the Mediterranean diet is the best medicine available to us to prevent disease and to live a long and healthy life.

Al: How can food be a medicine?

Emi: Food, like everything around us, is made up of chemical compounds. When we ingest food, our body breaks it down into tiny molecules that perform the functions we need to sustain life. If we eat the wrong foods or inadequate amounts, we create an unbalance in our body that in time can lead to disease.

Al: I had no idea food could have such an effect in our body.

Emi: Always keep in mind that our cells do their job with the material we supply them. Remember the old saying, "We are what we eat"?

Al: Yes.

What Type of "Fuel" Do You Feed Your Body?

Emi: Tell me something. What type of gasoline do you put in your car?

Al: Super. The best kind—which also happens to be the most expensive.

Emi: Any reason why you buy that kind of gas instead of buying the least expensive? You could save a lot of money.

Al: In the short run yes, but the engine runs more efficiently with high-quality fuel. Besides, the parts deteriorate much faster when you use cheap fluids. In the long run, I actually save money.

Emi: Do you use the same logic when you buy food at the market?

Al (*Looking surprised*): Well, that's not the same thing.

Emi: But it is. Like your car, your body is a machine made of different parts and your heart is the engine. The "fuel" you use to keep your heart and other body parts running makes a difference in your performance, whether it's at work, at school, with your family, or anywhere else. It also affects the speed at which your parts deteriorate.

Al (*Still showing astonishment*): Well, I guess it makes sense, the way you put it.

Emi: Actually, nowadays nutrition experts all over the world are making an effort to introduce the principles of the Mediterranean diet because centuries of experience have proved that it's the best "fuel" available to keep our "parts" running well until old age. Even the European community is recommending this healthy diet to all its members.

Al: Very interesting.

Emi: But the Mediterranean diet is more than just utilizing certain ingredients or recipes, which without a doubt contribute to our good health. A centuries-old tradition, this diet can only be understood when some of the customs and lifestyles of Mediterranean people are taken into account. In this region, people look forward to share meals with family and friends. Meals are a time to enjoy good tasty food while conversing, and sharing opinions and ideas—a time to relax.

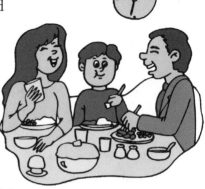

Al: I like to eat with family and friends.

Emi: That's excellent. Eating should not be a biological act done in a rush, its only purpose to fill up our stomachs. In fact, taking our time during meals is a proven healthy measure.

Al: I know I'm guilty of eating in a hurry many times, but I have so much work to do, I need to go back to my desk as soon as possible.

Emi: How much time do you get for lunch?

Al: One hour.

Emi: Do you usually take the whole hour for lunch, or do you go back to work before your time is up?

Al: I eat as fast as I can because my employees need me back.

Emi: I have no doubt they need you. But remember that all those things you have to do aren't going anywhere. Neither are your employees. I'm positive your company would love to see you take your whole time for lunch and relax for a little while before going back to work. When you do that, your level of productivity increases, and isn't that what a company wants?

Al (*Dead silence for a few seconds*): Is it true that people in the Mediterranean countries take a *siesta* [short nap] after lunch?

Emi: Yes.

Slow Down Your Heart with a *Siesta*

Emi: Most people in the Mediterranean countries don't like to rush through a meal. Eating in good company gives them an excuse to relax while dissecting current events or catching up with gossip. When possible, they also like to take a siesta.

Al: It sounds so relaxing.

Emi: It is. Scientific studies have associated good health not only with the ingestion of healthy foods but with a lifestyle linked to family life, lei-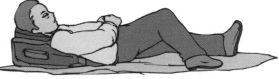sure time, regular physical activity, and traditional habits, such as taking a siesta.

Al: I wish I had the time to take a nap after lunch!

Emi: A siesta doesn't have to be two hours long. According to doctors, a 10- or 15-minute nap at midday helps to keep stress at bay. As a matter of fact, if you take a nap longer than 20 minutes, you may wake up with a headache and a general feeling of discomfort. How about if you take 15 minutes after you are done eating and have a snooze?

Al: I'll see what I can do, but I can't promise anything. You also mentioned physical activity. Does that mean I have to go to the gym?

Emi: Not unless you want to. People in Mediterranean countries don't have to go to the gym because physical activity is part of their daily life. Many scientific studies have shown that good nutrition and regular physical activity go hand and hand with the prevention and management of heart disease. During our discussions, we'll see how physical activity is a must to prevent and control high blood pressure, cholesterol, and triglycerides.

Al: What is so good about the Mediterranean diet?

Emi: It provides many benefits. Among them are the following:
- Daily physical activity
- Adequate amount of calories
- A diet high in fruits and vegetables
- Right proportion of healthy fats
- A diet low in sweets containing concentrated sugar

• Adequate intake of fiber and protein

• Adequate amounts of vitamins and minerals

A study conducted in Greece to investigate the survival rate among people with heart disease who followed the Mediterranean diet showed that based on a scale of 1 to 10, the people who adhered to the Mediterranean diet even by just 2 units had a 31 percent lower mortality rate from heart attacks than people who didn't follow the diet.[2] Studies have also shown that the combined effect of the Mediterranean diet, which includes physical activity, moderate alcohol use, and nonsmoking, is associated with a 50 percent lower risk of all-cause mortality.[3]

Al: That's a lot!

Emi: Yes. Now, I would like to take some time to learn about your eating habits. Can you take me through a typical day in your life?

Al: Sure! My meal patterns are very normal and don't change that much during the week.

Emi: Very well. Let's take a look.

Al's Typical Daily Diet

Emi: What do you usually have when you get up?

Al: A cup of coffee.

Emi: Caffeinated?

Al: Yes.

Emi: Do you put something in your coffee?

Al: Milk and 2 teaspoons of sugar.

Emi: What type of milk?

Al: Regular.

Emi: Do you take anything else before going to work?

Al: Yes. I have breakfast with my wife.

Emi: What do you eat?

Al: Most times my wife prepares a croissant sandwich with scrambled eggs and a couple of breakfast sausages for each of us. Sometimes we may have donuts or cereal.

Emi: What type of cereal?

Al: Corn flakes or something similar.

Emi: Do you drink something with your breakfast?

Al: A cup of coffee.

Emi: Do you have anything to eat or drink during the morning?

Al: I take a break around 10:00 and have a cup of coffee.

Emi: Do you eat lunch at work?

Al: I eat at the plant cafeteria. Most times I have a sandwich.

Emi: What kind of sandwich?

Al: I usually have some type of bologna like ham or turkey.

Emi: How many slices of meat do you use in your sandwich?

Al: Two. I also put a couple of cheese slices, and mayonnaise and mustard.

Emi: Anything else with your sandwich?

Al: Yes, a bag of potato chips.

Emi: What type of bread do you use for your sandwich?

Al: White.

Emi: Any other type of meat at lunchtime?

Al: Sometimes I have teriyaki chicken.

Emi: Do you include some salad with your lunch?

Al: Not really.

Emi: How about dessert?

Al: I usually grab some cookies or a piece of apple pie.

Emi: Do you eat fruit with your meal?

Al: Occasionally. I don't have time to eat fruit.

Emi: Anything to drink with your lunch?

Al: A soda.

Emi: What kind?

Al: Regular.

Emi: Do you eat or drink something in the afternoon?

Al: No.

Emi: What do you have for dinner?

Al: Depends. When my wife cooks, I like to have a piece of meat with French fries. We also have some vegetables—green beans or broccoli. When she works evenings the children and I may have a frozen dinner.

Emi: Do you have some salad with your dinner?

Al: Here and there.

Emi: Bread?

Al: Yes.

Emi: What kind?

Al: White.

Emi: What do you drink with your dinner?

Al: A soda. The children like soda.

Emi: Do you drink milk?

Al: With my coffee or when I have cereal.

Emi: Do you like yogurt?

Al: Yes. In the evenings I may also have some ice cream.

Emi: Thank you for the information. It will be very helpful in our search for solutions as we work together. (*Closing Al's file and putting it aside*) Today we are going to stop here. Do you have any questions about what we have covered today?

Al: No, but can you give me an overview of what you are going to cover in our meetings?

Emi: During the next three weeks we'll talk about the pillars of the Mediterranean diet and its benefits in relation to heart disease. It will give you a comprehensive view of how people in the Mediterranean countries have warded off this disease for centuries

Al: When you say "pillars," what are you referring to?

Emi: I'm referring to the components of this diet.

The Pillars of the Mediterranean Diet:

- Physical activity
- Fruits and vegetables
- Olive oil
- Legumes and whole grains
- Aromatic herbs, garlic, and onions

Al: Thank you. I'll be looking forward to our meetings. Are we meeting again on Wednesday as we established on the phone?

Emi: Yes. We'll meet three times a week, Mondays, Wednesdays, and Fridays for the next three weeks. Is 4:00 P.M. a convenient time for you?

Al: Yes, it's perfect because I leave work at 3:00 P.M.

Emi: Excellent. During our sessions I'll provide you with some written material for you to take home, but please bring a notebook because you may want to take notes as we speak.

Al: Sure. Is that all?

Emi: That's all. I'll see you on Wednesday. Have a great evening.

Al: The same to you.

REFERENCES

1. The EPIC (European Prospective Investigation into Cancer and Nutrition) Study, http://www.iarc.fr/epic/; PREDIMED (Prevención con Dieta Mediterránea) Study, www.predimed.org.

2. Trichopoulou A, Bamia C, Trichopoulos D. Mediterranean diet and survival among patients with coronary heart disease in Greece. *Archives of Internal Medicine.* 2005 Apr 25;165(8):929–35.

3. Knoops KT, de Groot LC, Kromhout D, Perrin AE, Moreiras-Varela O, Menotti A, van Staveren WA. Mediterranean diet, lifestyle factors, and 10-year mortality in elderly European men and women: the HALE project. *Journal of the American Medical Association.* 2004 Sep 22;292(12):1433–9.

Chapter Two

Physical Activity: A Magical Pill

Counseling Session—Day 2
Wednesday, 4:00 P.M.

Emi: Good afternoon, Al. It is nice to see you again. How was traffic today?

Al: No major traffic jams.

Emi: Do you need a few minutes to relax?

Al: No, we can go ahead. I brought a notebook as you indicated.

Emi: Very good. Let's start then. Today we are going to see how being physically active is the best treatment we can give our hearts.

Al: I thought our discussions would be on the components of the Mediterranean diet.

Emi: They will. That's why we are talking about physical activity today, because it's one of the most important ingredients in this diet. In fact, without physical activity, there is no Mediterranean diet.

Al: I see.

Emi: Do you walk regularly?

Al: What do you mean?

Emi: Do you go for a walk most days of the week?

13

Al: No. I don't have the time to walk.

Emi: If I told you there is a "magical pill" that lowers cholesterol and triglycerides, helps prevent and control high blood pressure, reduces feelings of stress, improves mental health, and gives you more energy, would you take it?

Al: Sure. Make it two.

Emi (*Showing Al a pair of walking shoes*): Well, here are your pills.

Al (*Looking puzzled, then laughing*): A little hard to swallow, don't you think?

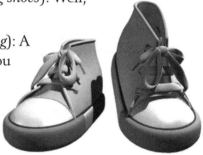

Emi: Not at all. As you might have guessed, the "magical pill" is physical activity.

Al (*Recovering from his fit of laughter*): That was funny!

Emi: Well, before 1900, very few people died of heart attacks in the United States; since then, however, heart disease has become the number one killer.

Al: What has changed since then?

Emi: Very simple. The age of technology has made life very easy for all of us. Before the Industrial Revolution, nobody went to the gym; most people made their living through some sort of manual labor, and walking was the major means of transportation. With the arrival of automation, life has become less strenuous and most manual labor has been either replaced or assisted by machinery.

Al: Yes, you are right. Modern conveniences have made physical activity unnecessary.

Emi: In addition, with this change in lifestyle came a change in diet: hamburgers, French fries, and large sodas. This combination of a sedentary life and a diet rich in fat and sugar has led to an increase in clogged blood vessels.

Al: What do you mean by "sedentary"?

Emi: Inactive, not moving enough. Over the past 50 years, health professionals have examined the association between physical activity and the risk for heart disease. The findings consistently reveal that people who are physically active have half the risk for heart attacks than the people who are not active. Those studies show also that at least 30 minutes of moderate physical activity, such as brisk walking, on most days of the week, is sufficient to reduce the risk of heart attack.[1]

Al: (*Al makes some notes in his notebook*): Should I join a gym?

Walking Makes Your Heart Stronger

Emi: Only if you want to. The 1996 Report of the Surgeon General tells us that physical activity doesn't need to be strenuous to obtain health benefits.[2] Just walking, if done daily, can help lower your risk of heart disease because brisk walking is an aerobic exercise that conditions the heart and the lungs. The overall evidence of some studies reviewed by Dr. Wannamethee and colleagues on the effect moderate physical activity has on heart disease showed that it doesn't have to be vigorous or sports-related to achieve results. The studies also support the recommended guidelines of 30 minutes of moderate physical activity on most days of the week as prevention.[3] Similar findings come from a review carried out by Haennel et al., where the researchers concluded that moderate activity, such as brisk walking for 30 to 60 minutes a day most days of the week, is associated with significant reductions in deaths caused by heart attacks.[4]

Al: The results of these studies seem to be consistent.

Emi: Yes. We have to keep in mind that the heart is a muscle, and like any other muscle in the body, it becomes stronger the more we exercise it. A strong heart can pump more blood with fewer beats and less effort, thus putting less strain on the blood vessels. This translates into lower blood pressure.

Al: I didn't know the heart is a muscle.

Emi: Not many people do, but without exercise, it loses muscle fibers and becomes weak until it is unable to do its job. And the last thing we need is a heart that cannot do its job.

Al: I can't agree more. How can physical activity lower the risk of heart disease?

Emi: In several ways. I will list them for you.

Direct Effects of Physical Activity on Heart Disease

- Makes the heart stronger so it can pump more blood with fewer beats.

- Lowers blood pressure by increasing the diameter of the *coronary arteries*, the arteries that wrap the heart, making them more elastic and forming new blood vessels. The researchers at the University of Connecticut tell us that the effect of exercise on hypertension is immediate. This effect is obtained by 30 minutes or more of continuous or accumulated physical activity per day.[5]

- Lowers LDL, the "bad" cholesterol. The Emory University School of Medicine in Atlanta conducted a study with 28 mice to investigate the effects of a diet with or without exercise on LDL cholesterol. The study showed that the group that was exercised had a lower level of LDL cholesterol and a lower level of damage in the arteries as compared to the group that did not exercise.[6]

- Increases the level of HDL, the "good" cholesterol. A study conducted by the Heart Institute in India showed that physical activity, consisting mostly of a 60-minute morning walk each day, was associated with a rise in HDL cholesterol, the "good" guy, in patients who had a heart attack.[7]

- Decreases triglycerides. Triglycerides can get deposited on the lining of arteries, a factor that leads to clogging.

- Decreases the risk of *diabetes*, which is a risk for heart attack.

- Reduces the amount of *platelets*, tiny disks in the blood, which reduces the risk for clog formation.

Al: Wow! I was physically active when I was young. Do you think that would help with my cholesterol?

Emi: No. People who are very active during their youth but then become sedentary lose most of the benefits they acquired during that period of their life. One of the reasons people in the Mediterranean countries have one of lowest incidence of heart disease in the world is because they are active throughout their whole lives.

Al (*Lolling back in the comfortable armchair*): Well, these studies are convincing, but I don't have the time to be physically active.

Do You Have Time to Be Physically Active?

Emi: You don't have to go to the gym if you don't want to or if you can't find the time, but you can be physically active during the day if you become aware of the opportunities available to you. Actually, the best recipe you can try to lower cholesterol and high blood pressure is to do what Mediterranean people do: walk.

Al: But where do they walk?

Emi: They walk to the subway, to the bus, to the movies, to the restaurant, to the store, to the bank. They go out with family and friends. Do you know that according to the North Central Texas Council of Governments, 75 percent of the trips taken by car in the United States are less than 1 mile?

Al: I saw something to that regard in a movie. It was hilarious.

Emi: It may sound funny, but the sad reality is that physical inactivity is linked to deaths caused by heart attacks.

Al: You are right; I should not laugh at something so serious. But as I said before, although this is convincing, I don't have time to walk.

Emi: I'm sure if we look carefully at your daily schedule we can find some room for some physical activity.

Al: I doubt it. I'm a very busy person.

Emi: Let's give a try.

Finding the Time to Walk

Emi: How big is your company's parking lot?

Al: Pretty big.

Emi: Where do you park?

Al: I have an assigned parking space close to the main entrance.

Emi: Why close to the entrance?

Al: It's part of a manager's fringe benefits.

Emi: Can you ask your supervisor to assign you a parking space at the farthest corner of the parking lot?

Al (*Looking dumbfounded*): Why would I want to do that?

Emi: So you can walk. You can leave home 10 minutes earlier and walk from your new assigned parking space to your office. When you leave work, you'll have to walk back to your car for another 10 minutes. By doing this, you will have walked 20 minutes every business day, provided you don't ask a co-worker to give you a ride to your car, of course.

Al: People in my company are going to think I'm nuts.

Emi: Let them think whatever they want, as long as your cholesterol and blood pressure go down. If you tell them what you're doing they might even want to join you.

Al: Alright, I'll talk to human resources, but I'm afraid they may think I'm losing it.

Emi: I doubt it. Also, when you go to the movies, to the mall, or anyplace else, do the same: park as far as you can from the entrance. Don't circle the parking lot over and over in search of a parking spot by the entrance. By parking far away you keep adding minutes to your walking without interfering with your daily schedule. What do you do during TV commercials?

Al: I change channels.

Emi: You could walk instead.

Al: Where?

Emi: In your living room.

Al *(Rolling his eyes)*: I won't get too far walking there!

Emi: You can walk quite a bit in your living room by pacing back and forth. A two-hour movie will give you probably between 30 and 40 minutes of commercials. You can also try jumping jacks.

Make Your Dog Your Walking Partner

Emi: Do you have a dog?

Al: Yes, Napoleon.

Emi: That's an interesting name.

Al: When we got him, my son Greg was taking a French history class and he insisted on naming him Napoleon.

Emi: Do you walk him?

Al: Sometimes.

Emi: How often is "sometimes"?

Al: Once a week.

Emi: How does he get his exercise the rest of the week?

Al: He plays in the backyard with a ball. That's all he needs.

Emi: Do you know that nowadays many dogs are dying at an early age because of lack of exercise?

Al: No, I didn't.

Emi: Dogs need to walk, just as people do. When they don't, they accumulate cholesterol in their arteries and they can die of a heart attack. How about walking with your dog 15 or 20 minutes every day? It would benefit both of you.

Al: Okay, I'll walk the dog. I hope he appreciates what I am doing for him!

Emi: He will; dogs are very grateful. And bear in mind that any duration of physical activity counts, whether it's 15 minutes, or 15 hours; whether you take a walk during lunch break or you ride all day in the Tour de France. Over the course of a day, brief bouts of activity can add up to a lot of exercise. Walking up the stairs at home also counts as exercise, as well as dusting your living room or using your vacuum cleaner. One of the important points Surgeon General Donna Shalala made in her 1996 report on Physical Activity and Health was that any exercise helps and that the total amount of physical activity can be cumulative.

Stairs for a Strong Heart

Emi: One of the best exercises you can do to make your heart stronger is to use stairs. If your office is on the sixth floor, leave the elevator on the second or third floor and walk the remaining flights.

Al: My office is on the first floor.

Emi: How many stories do you have in your office building?

Al: Eight.

Emi: Well, how about if you ask a coworker to walk with you up the stairs at lunchtime? Before you know it, you may have a group joining you and it could be a lot of fun. You could use this time to catch up with the office gossip and by the time you go home, you would have covered 30 to 40 minutes of physical activity without interfering with the rest of your daily tasks.

Al: That gossip business is not a bad idea. I have been so busy I am falling behind on it.

Emi: Do you have stairs at home?

Al: Yes, our house has two stories.

Emi: Take things up the stairs one at a time instead of letting them pile up for one trip. How about dancing, do you like it?

Al: Yes.

Emi: Does your wife like it also?

Al: Yes. You know, that's a good idea! I know a place where they have free salsa classes, and people can stay afterwards for the dancing. I'll ask my wife if she wants to go. She is always complaining because we don't go out enough.

Emi: Excellent! How would you feel about taking the whole family for an outing in the mountains one of these Sundays?

Al: I don't think the children will go for it. They are always doing something with their friends or in their room with the computer and games. I barely see them.

Emi: Try. You will never know unless you ask. Have you ever used a pedometer?

Al: What is that?

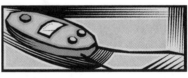

Emi (*Showing him the pedometer on top of the table*): A step counter. It's a good way to check how much you walk during the day. Time yourself every time you walk, go up and down stairs, vacuum your carpet, or wash your car. You might be surprised at how many steps you may have accumulated by the end of the day. You can get a pedometer at any sporting goods store.

Al: I'll get one this weekend. How many steps a day do I need to show on the pedometer to make walking meaningful?

Emi: Health authorities recommend 10,000 steps but even 5,000 is a good number. You don't have to run a marathon or climb the Himalayas to achieve fitness.

Al: That's a relief because I suffer from fear of heights. I told my wife what you said Monday about the Mediterranean diet and she is interested in learning more about it. She's worried about me and wants to help in any way she can.

Emi: Of course, that's understandable. Tell her she is welcome to come with you to our meetings. Many of the lifestyle changes you will need to make will affect the whole family and if she is familiar with those changes, the transition will be much easier for everyone. In fact, the changes will benefit the whole family.

Al: I hope so. I am also worried that some of the factors that have caused my health condition could also be affecting her and the children.

Emi: You are right. Lack of physical activity and the wrong diet can wreak havoc with our bodies. That's why no amount of cure can replace prevention.

Al: Yeah, you are right. I'll tell my wife about your invitation, but unfortunately her daily hours make it impossible for her to come. Thank you very much. (*Looking at his watch*) I think our time is up. Are we done for the day?

Emi: Yes, unless you have any questions.

Al: No, I don't. I'll see you Friday.

Emi: Have a wonderful evening.

REFERENCES

1. Thompson P. Preventing coronary heart disease. The role of physical activity. *The Physician and Sportsmedicine*. 2001 Feb;29(2).

2. A Report of the Surgeon General: Physical Activity and Health. 1996. U.S. Department of Health and Human Services.

3. Wannamethee SG, Shaper AG. Physical activity and cardiovascular disease. *Seminars Vascular Medicine*. 2002 Aug;2(3):257–66.

4. Haennel RG, Lemire F. Physical activity to prevent cardiovascular disease. How much is enough? *Canadian Family Physician*. 2002 Jan;48:65–71.

5. Pescatello LS. Exercise and hypertension: recent advances in exercise prescription. *Current Hypertension Reports*. 2005 Aug;7(4):281–6.

6. Ramachandran S, Penumetcha M, Merchant NK, Santanam N, Roug R, Parthasarathy S. Exercise reduces preexisting atherosclerotic lesions in LDL receptor knock out mice. *Atherosclerosis*. 2005 Jan;178(1):33–8.

7. Mukherjee M, Shetty KR. Variations in high-density lipoprotein cholesterol in relation to physical activity and Taq 1B polymorphism of the cholesterol ester transfer protein gene. *Clinical Genetics*. 2004 May;65(5):412–8.

Chapter Three

The Sinister Connection: High Blood Pressure and Processed Foods

Counseling Session—Day 3
Friday, 4:00 P.M.

Al: I have good news for you.

Emi: Fantastic! I can use some today.

Al: The human resources department has assigned me one of the farthest spaces in the company's parking lot.

Emi: That's excellent news, Al! What did they say when you asked them?

Al: They thought it was great. They are going to write an article in the company's newsletter telling the story.

Emi: You are going to be very popular.

Al: Looks like it. I also walked Napoleon last night.

Emi: You did? Where did you take him?

Al: We strolled for about 30 minutes in the neighborhood. He seemed to be really happy, especially when he met other doggies during the outing.

Emi: And he will be much healthier if you continue to walk him.

Al: I will. I really love my dog, and I don't want him to die of a heart attack. I want him to be with us for a long time.

Emi: I am very glad it worked so well for the two of you. This is definitely good news. Are you ready to start?

Al: Yes.

Emi: Today we're going to talk about high blood pressure.

Al: My doctor mentioned the word *hypertension* during my visit to his office. What exactly is it?

Emi: Hypertension is the medical term for high blood pressure.

Al: I see. And what is high blood pressure?

What Is High Blood Pressure, or Hypertension?

Emi: Blood pressure is how forcefully the blood is banging against the walls of the arteries. If you have high blood pressure it means the heart is pounding harder than it should to send through the blood vessels the nutrients and oxygen the cells need to maintain life.

Al: Is high blood pressure life threatening?

Emi: Very much! As you probably know, the heart never stops working; it pumps blood to the whole body seven days a week, twenty-four hours a day.

Al: How exhausting!

Emi: Indeed! Continuous high blood pressure causes the walls of the *arteries* to thicken, a condition that reduces the blood flow. It also makes the inside of

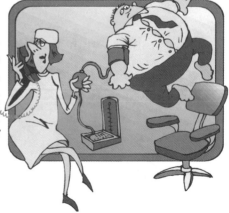

the arteries rough, contributing to the formation of *plaque*, mounds of fat and debris deposited in the wall of arteries. Plaque reduces the space available for blood to circulate, which means the already hardworking heart has to work even harder to send blood to the cells through narrowed blood vessels.

Al: Oh my!

Emi: Actually, it can get worse because a heart that has to work strenuously for long periods of time becomes enlarged. A slightly distended heart may function properly, but a severely enlarged heart must work with all its might to pump blood through the blood vessels. If the condition persists, the heart and blood vessels may get further damaged, increasing the risk of a stroke or a heart attack. People with uncontrolled high blood pressure are three times more likely to develop heart disease, and seven times more likely to have a stroke.

Al: You were right; it did get worse.

Emi: Hypertension may also lead to other serious complications.

Al: There's more?

Additional Complications of High Blood Pressure

Emi: Over time, increased pressure on the inner walls of blood vessels can weaken them and form an *aneurysm*, the ballooning of the artery. This ballooning may cause the blood vessel to rupture, resulting in internal bleeding. Bleeding into the brain or the spaces surrounding it, causes a *hemorrhagic stroke*. Hypertension is by far the most potent risk factor for stroke.

Al: Good heavens! What do I need to do to keep my blood pressure down?

Emi: You have to fight this war on several fronts:
- Be physically active. People who are not physically active are 30 to 50 percent more likely to develop hypertension.
- Limit *sodium* in your diet.

- Don't smoke.
- Avoid high alcohol consumption; 5 to 7 percent of the hypertension we see in people is due to high alcohol intake.
- Avoid stress.
- Maintain an appropriate body weight.

Al: What exactly is sodium?

Emi: Salt is made up of two minerals—sodium and chloride. Sodium is the part in salt that can be bad for our health and the one we find listed on food labels. About half of the salt we eat is sodium.

Al: What is wrong with sodium? Why is it such a problem?

Why Is Sodium a Problem?

Emi: Sodium is a problem because wherever sodium goes, water goes. Since both are inseparable, when we eat a lot of salt we retain a large volume of fluid in our blood vessels that needs to be moved around. And what do you think moves all that fluid in our body?

Al: The heart?

Emi: Exactly. On the other hand, when we reduce the amount of salt in our diets, our cells don't hang on to so much water, the heart does not have to work so hard, and our blood pressure goes down. According to Meneton, from an evolutionary viewpoint, the human species is adapted to ingest and excrete less than 1 gram (1,000 milligrams) of salt per day, an amount 10 times lower than the average values observed in industrialized countries. The study showed that salt increases the thickness and stiffness of the arteries, increasing the incidence of strokes and the severity of heart attacks.[1]

Al: You know, I was caught by surprise when my doctor told me I have high blood pressure. How can I have high blood pressure and not know?

Emi: Because high blood pressure has no symptoms.

High Blood Pressure: "The Silent Killer"

Emi: In most cases, hypertension has no warning signs and it causes no symptoms until it reaches a life-threatening stage. People usually find out their blood pressure is high through a routine visit to the doctor, as you did. In fact, hypertension is known as "the silent killer." Very severe hypertension may cause dizziness, headaches, nausea, or vomiting, but this is rare. High blood pressure is one of the major health problems of the 21st century. According to Elijah Saunders, M.D., professor at the University of Maryland School of Medicine, cardiologist and hypertension expert, "only about half of the people in this country who have high blood pressure know they have it. Of those who know they have it, only about half are being treated for it. And of those being treated, only about half actually have their blood pressure under control."[2]

Al: That's scary! When we talk about high blood pressure, how high is high?

How High Is High?

Emi: High blood pressure is defined as a blood pressure greater than 140 over 90. Optimal blood pressure in an adult is 120/80 mm HG (millimeters of mercury), although it can range from 110/70 to 140/90. Physicians use two measurements to describe blood pressure:

- *Systolic blood pressure.* It is measured as the heart contracts to send blood out into the blood vessels. It is the first number in the reading, the high one.
- *Diastolic blood pressure.* It is measured as the heart relaxes to allow blood to come back into the heart. It is the second number in the reading, the low one. You can see the different classifications of blood pressure in this table (*see next page*).

Al: I should watch the amount of sodium I consume?

Emi: Yes.

Al: How do I do that?

TABLE #2—BLOOD PRESSURE CLASSIFICATION

Category	Systolic (mm Hg)	Diastolic (mm Hg)
Optimal	less than 120	less than 80
Normal	less than 130	less than 85
High normal	130–139	85–89
Hypertension		
Stage 1	140–159	90–99
Stage 2	160–179	100–109
Stage 3	180 and above	110 and above

Table #2— From the Sixth Report of the Joint National Committee on Detection, Evaluation, and Treatment of High Blood Pressure.

Emi: By cutting down on processed foods and loading up on fruits and vegetables.

Al: What is the highest amount of sodium I can have on a daily basis without causing harm to my arteries?

How Much Sodium Can You Have?

Emi: For years, the standard recommendation was a diet that limited sodium intake to no more than 2,400 milligrams per day. However, the findings from the DASH-Sodium trial found that lower intakes are even more beneficial. The DASH study found that an intake of 1,500 milligrams a day produced the biggest blood pressure reduction when being part of a diet low in saturated fat and cholesterol as well as an adequate intake of fruits and vegetables.[3] We also know that hypertension rarely occurs in countries in which people consume less than 1,000 milligrams of sodium per day.

Al: How much salt is 1,500 milligrams?

Emi: Here is a table to guide you with sodium equivalents.

TABLE #3—SODIUM EQUIVALENTS

Amount of Salt	Equivalent Amount of Sodium (milligrams)
¼ teaspoon salt	600 mg sodium
½ teaspoon salt	1,200 mg sodium
⅔ teaspoon salt	1,500 mg sodium
¾ teaspoon salt	1,800 mg sodium
1 teaspoon salt (6 grams of salt)	2,400 mg sodium

Al: How can I keep sodium that low?

Emi: By lowering the amount of processed foods you eat and increasing the amount of fruits and vegetables in your diet. Processed foods are very high in sodium.

Al: Why are they so high in sodium?

Emi: Manufacturers of processed foods use salt as a preventive measure because salt keeps *microbes*—microscopic organisms that transmit disease—at bay.

Al: Are there any specific processed foods I need to stay away from?

Emi: I am tempted to say all of them, but since we have to be realistic, let us see what you can do to minimize sodium in your diet.

Sodium and Processed Foods

Emi: Always keep in mind that about 75 percent of the salt we eat every day comes from processed foods, most of which is added by food manufacturers and restaurants; 15 percent comes from cooking and 10 percent from natural foods. Because the American public consumes far more sodium than is needed, about 4,000 milligrams per day, on November 2002 the American Public Health Association called for a

50 percent reduction in sodium in the nation's food supply over the next 10 years. It's estimated that such a reduction would save at least 150,000 lives annually.[4]

Al: That's a lot of lives!

Emi: A lot! I want you to become familiar with reading food labels. The first place to start when you look at the nutrition facts label is the serving size and the number of servings in the package. Then ask yourself how many servings you are consuming: ½, 1, 2, and so forth. The serving size is important because if the package provides two servings and you eat the whole box, you are doubling the daily percentage values you ingest.

Nutrition Facts		
Serving Size 1 Package (227g)		
Amount Per Serving		
Calories 270	Calories from Fat 140	
		% Daily Value*
Total Fat 16g		**24%**
Saturated Fat 6g		**32%**
Cholesterol 55mg		**19%**
Sodium 1380mg		**57%**
Total Carbohydrate 20g		**7%**
Dietary Fiber 2g		**7%**
Sugars 3g		
Protein 11g		
Vitamin A 8%	•	Vitamin C 8%
Calcium 6%	•	Iron 8%

*Percent Daily Values are based on a 2,000 calorie diet. Your daily values may be higher or lower depending on your calorie needs.

	Calories:	2,000	2,500
Total Fat	Less than	65g	80g
Saturated Fat	Less than	20g	25g
Cholesterol	Less than	300mg	300mg
Sodium	Less than	2,400mg	2,400mg
Total Carbohydrate		300g	375g
Dietary Fiber		25g	30g

Calories per gram:
Fat 9 • Carbohydrate 4 • Protein 4

Al: I see the amount of sodium in this package is almost the total amount I should eat during the whole day. This means it's very high, isn't it?

Emi: Extremely high. I'm glad you noticed it. If you buy processed foods, look for products that have "no salt added" or are low in sodium, 140 milligrams or less per serving. A rule of thumb is not to eat more than 500 milligrams of sodium per meal. Pay special attention to the following items because they can be high in sodium:

- Frozen entrées
- Canned vegetables, soups, and sauces
- Lunch meats such as bologna, ham, turkey, or smoked salmon
- Pickled foods

- Instant breakfast cereals, frozen biscuits
- Snack items such as salted nuts, pretzels, chips, and crackers
- Fast foods
- Cheese
- Bread

Al: I must confess all this is new to me. I never bothered looking at food labels.

Emi: That's very common. Many people are not aware of how much information we can obtain from a food label.

Al: How am I doing with the sodium in my diet?

Emi: Not very well. It's quite high.

Al: What am I eating that makes it so high?

Emi: Let's take a look.

TABLE #4—AL'S USUAL DIET

Food Description	Measure	Sodium (mg)
Breakfast		
Eggs	2	126
Turkey breakfast sausage	2	376
Cereal, corn flakes	1 cup	300
Croissant	1	424
Milk, 1% low fat	1 cup	123
Total sodium at breakfast time		1,349
Lunch		
Bologna, turkey	2 slices	492
American cheese	2 slices	800
Wheat bread	2 slices	266
Mustard, prepared	1 packet = 1 tsp	126
Mayo type, regular	1 tbsp	214
Potato chips	1 bag	119
Apple pie, 1/6 of pie	1 piece	444
Total sodium at lunch time		2,461
Total sodium breakfast and lunch		**3,810**

Al: Good Lord! I won't be able to eat anything from now on!

Emi: Yes you will. Let's explore what items you can replace to lower sodium and still enjoy your meals:

- Replace the croissant with 100 percent whole grain bread.
- Replace the sausages with a piece of fruit.
- Replace corn flakes with oatmeal. Try Organic Old Fashioned Oatmeal Hot Cereal from Arrowhead Mills. It has no sodium, and as we'll see when we talk about grains, oatmeal contains the type of fiber that lowers cholesterol.

Al: That sounds good.

Emi: Do you think you may enjoy this breakfast?

Al: To be honest with you, not as much as the old one. This is a big change, but I am willing to make it. I know that having my arteries clogged is a serious business, and I don't want to grow old and be crippled with heart disease.

Emi: That is an excellent attitude, and it's going to help you very much. Let me show you how your new breakfast would look.

TABLE #5—AL'S NEW BREAKFAST

Food Description	Measure	Sodium (mg)
Breakfast #1		
Scrambled eggs	2	126
100% whole grain bread, low sodium	2	8
Fruit (apple, banana, orange, pineapple, etc.)	1 piece	2
Coffee with some milk	1 cup	30
Total sodium breakfast #1		**166**
Breakfast #2		
Old Fashioned Oatmeal Hot Cereal	½ cup	0
Milk, 1% low fat, added to hot cereal	½ cup	123
Fruit (apple, blueberries, strawberries, etc)	1 piece	2
Total sodium breakfast #2		**125**

Al: Gee, that's quite a difference in the amount of sodium!

Emi: Yes. Now let's look at ways to reduce some of the sodium in your lunch:

- Avoid cold cuts and hard processed cheeses. Replace them with chicken breast or fish.
- Eliminate salty potato chips. Replace them with rice or pasta.
- Order a salad.
- Order a vegetable side dish.
- Include a piece of fruit.

Al: Can I order chicken teriyaki?

Emi: Teriyaki sauce is very high in sodium. One 4.5-ounce teriyaki chicken breast has about 1,866 milligrams of sodium.

Al: You're kidding!

Emi: No, I'm not. Stay away from it.

Al: What can I use in place of salt when I cook?

Emi: You can use herbs, garlic, spices, lemon, lime, and vinegar. Use extra virgin olive oil and lemon or vinegar for your salads. Do not buy salt substitutes; they are very high in potassium, way over the amount the body needs.

Al: I suspect I will need to take a calculator with me when I go to the market.

Emi: You don't have to if you stay away from processed foods as much as possible and do the bulk of your shopping at the produce section. Fruits and vegetables are very low in sodium. In fact, the sodium content of a piece of fruit ranges from 0 to 5 milligrams and from 1 to 70 milligrams in vegetables.

Al: That's low. Then, based on what you're saying, fruits and vegetables help lower blood pressure?

Emi: Correct! Let's take a break. When we come back we'll talk about how fruits and vegetables can fight blood pressure.

REFERENCES

1. Meneton P, Jeunemaitre X, E. de Wardener H, Macgregor G. Links between dietary salt intake, renal salt handling, blood pressure, and cardiovascular diseases. *Physiological Reviews*. 2005;85:679–715.

2. Saunders E, M.D. High blood pressure: tips to stop the silent killer. University of Maryland, Medical Center. By Noel Holton, University of Maryland Medical System Web Site Writer.

3. "Dietary Approaches to Stop Hypertension" (DASH) clinical study. National Heart, Lung, and Blood Institute (NHLBI) and National Institutes of Health. Results appeared April 17, 1997, issue of the *New England Journal of Medicine*. Available at: http://www.nih.gov/news/pr/apr97/Dash.htm.

4. Havas S, Rocella E, Lenfant C. Reducing the public health burden from elevated blood pressure levels in the United States by lowering intake of dietary sodium. *American Journal of Public Health*. 2004 Jan;Vol 94, N.1, 19–22.

Chapter Four

Fruits and Vegetables: Your Heart's Friends

Counseling Session—Day 3 (Continuation)
Friday, after the break

Emi: Do you like fruit?

Al: Yes. But I am not in the habit of eating it.

Emi: Well, the latest research shows that the biggest payoff from eating fruits and vegetables is for the heart.

Al: Because they can lower high blood pressure?

Emi: And much more, as we'll see.

The Sodium-Potassium Balance

Emi: We have seen that sodium content in fruits ranges from 0 to 5 milligrams per serving. That means if you eat four pieces of fruit a day, you are ingesting only 20 milligrams of sodium. Vegetables range from 1 to 70 milligrams. An average portion of vegetables contains about 10 milligrams of sodium thus, four portions of vegetables amount to about 40 milligrams. At the same time, when you eat fruits and vegetables, you are replacing other foods in your meals that may be high in sodium.

35

Al: I guess you can't beat that. Now I understand why you told me to do most of my shopping in the produce section.

Emi: Exactly. But fruits and vegetables contribute much more to the fight against heart disease than being low in sodium. For example, they are high in *potassium.*

Al: What is potassium?

Emi: Potassium is a mineral that plays a key role in heart functions and muscle contractions, making it an important nutrient for a normal heart. It works with sodium to regulate the water balance in the body. Diets low in sodium and high in potassium lower blood pressure, which reduces stroke risk.[1] Studies have shown that our diets should be five times higher in potassium than in sodium to maintain normal blood pressure. Unfortunately, in the typical American diet, the amount of sodium is five times higher than potassium. [Please consult with your doctor if you are taking potassium tablets.]

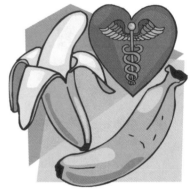

Al: How did we manage to get it so wrong?

Emi: By eating a diet high in processed foods and low in fruits and vegetables. Another benefit of eating fruits and vegetables is that they provide substantial amounts of *calcium* and *magnesium,* two minerals essential for a healthy heart and consistently associated with lower blood pressure.

Calcium, Magnesium, and Blood Pressure

Al: I thought only dairy products had calcium but you are saying that fruits and vegetables are also rich in this mineral?

Emi: Yes, especially green leafy vegetables.

Al: I know we need calcium for the bones, but I never heard of calcium being good for the heart.

Emi: Calcium is extremely important in maintaining normal blood pressure; it is required for nerve transmission and regulation of heart muscle function. Many studies have shown that as we increase the consumption of foods with a high content of calcium, the risk of high blood pressure decreases, especially if we maintain adequate intakes of magnesium.

Al: I am not familiar with magnesium either.

Emi: Magnesium is needed for more than 300 biochemical reactions in the body. Having adequate amounts of magnesium in our bodies helps the heart maintain a steady rhythm and normal blood pressure. Lately, medical science has been taking a close look at the role magnesium plays in preventing and managing health conditions such as hypertension and heart disease. Green leafy vegetables are good sources of magnesium because the center of the chlorophyll molecule, which gives green vegetables their color, contains magnesium.

Al: I understand. But my problem is that I don't have time to eat fruit.

Emi: Eating fruit doesn't have to be time-consuming; there are plenty of ways you can include fruit in your diet.

Al: How?

Fruit Instead of Cake

Emi: A practical way to include fruit in your diet is to have it as dessert. How does it sound to you to replace the cookies you have after lunch with a piece of fruit?

Al: Hm.

Emi: That's how people in the Mediterranean countries consume fruit most of the time. You know, my mother never allowed me to leave the table without eating a piece of fruit. She never had a supply of cookies at home, and we never ate cookies or cake for dessert except on special occasions, such as birthdays or holidays. Even then, I could have some cake only after I had eaten a piece of fruit.

Al: My mother never did that. She always had all sort of cookies in the pantry. Maybe that's why I am not used to eating fruit with my meals. In fact, most of the time we had cookies or pie for dessert at home.

Emi: That's a problem we see quite often in families. Nutrition experts are now warning us that the consumption of pastries is one of the reasons we see an epidemic of children with high cholesterol. The habit of eating foods high in salt and fat is acquired during childhood and is the cause of plaque at an early age. Talk to your wife and start including fruit in your main meals, either as dessert or in salads. It will benefit the whole family, and your children will get used to eating fruit as part of a healthy diet. They will be grateful when they are older because good eating habits can prevent many diseases.

Al: I like that thought very much.

Emi: In the meantime, try not to choose cookies or pie for dessert when you eat out. Order a piece of fresh fruit. You can also include fruit in your breakfast.

Al: How?

Add Fruit to Your Breakfast

Emi: For example, you can prepare a fruit shake, or smoothie. I always keep different kinds of organic berries in my freezer. In the morning, I put ½ cup of rice milk, ½ cup of plain nonfat yogurt, ¾ cup of frozen berries, and half a banana in the blender, and in a minute I have a delicious breakfast. Talk about fast food! If you prefer to use cow's milk, use 1 percent lowfat. Do you like fruit salads?

Al: I don't know; I never eat them.

Emi: I'll tell you how I prepare them. These are two of my favorites:

1. Cut small pieces of apples, bananas, oranges, and peaches. Splash fresh orange juice over the fruit and mix it. It tastes delicious.

2. Cut an apple and a few strawberries into small pieces—or any other fruit you like. Throw in 1 cup of plain nonfat yogurt, a few raisins, and six walnuts. It is out of this world.

Al: It sounds tasty.

Emi: Try to buy *organic* fruit if you can. The flavor of the fruit is sweeter.

Al: Where can I buy organic fruit?

Emi: Nowadays many supermarkets and farmers' markets carry a good selection of organic products. I like to support my local farmers' market, so I go there on Thursdays to do part of my grocery shopping. Check what day your local farmers' market is in your area and go with your children. It will be a great experience for them. And above all, keep in mind that you have to eat plenty of fruits and vegetables if you are serious about lowering your blood pressure.

Al: How much is plenty?

Emi: More than most people eat.

How Much Fruit Should You Eat?

Emi: The latest recommendations from health authorities call for four or five servings of fruit, depending on one's caloric intake. For example, if a person needs 2,000 calories a day, the appropriate number of servings would be four. [Note: If you have been diagnosed with diabetes do not eat more than three pieces of fruit a day.]

Al: I see. Earlier during our discussions you mentioned frozen fruit. I thought frozen fruit was less nutritious than fresh fruit.

Emi: It depends.

Fresh or Frozen?

Emi: There are times when frozen fruits and vegetables can be more nutritious than fresh. They are frozen immediately after they are picked, and many times the vitamins and minerals

are better preserved in frozen foods than in their fresh coun-
terpart, which need to be transported and stored for a long
time before they reach the store.

Al: That's good to know.

The Place for Vegetables in Our Diet

Emi: Let us talk now about vegetables.

Al: I don't care for vegetables. I was not born to be a vegetarian.

Emi: You don't have to be one, but make sure your diet includes
more plant foods than processed products and not the other
way around. The recommendations from health authorities
call for about five to seven servings of vegetables, depending
on one's caloric intake. For example, a person eating 2,000
calories a day should have five servings.

Al: How do I know what a serving is?

What Is a Serving?

FRUITS:
- A standard piece of fruit, the size of a regular light bulb
- ¼ cup dried fruit
- ½ cup fresh, frozen, or canned fruit
- 6 ounces fruit juice

VEGETABLES:
- 1 cup raw leafy vegetables
- ½ cup cooked vegetables
- 6 ounces vegetable juice

Emi: If you get into the habit of having a piece of fruit for dessert
with your three main meals you don't have to worry about
counting servings. And the same goes for vegetables. If you
make a salad and a vegetable side dish part of your lunch
and dinner you won't need to count vegetable servings either. If you are hungry during the day have a piece of fruit
such as an apple, banana, or peach.

Al: The problem with vegetables is that they are boring.

Emi: Well, that depends on how you prepare them. How do you cook vegetables at home?

Al: I boil them.

Emi: And then? How do you serve them?

Al: Just boiled.

Emi: That's why. Plain boiled vegetables can be quite boring.

Al: How do you prepare them?

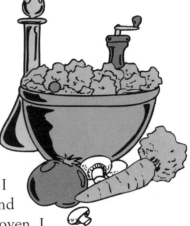

Emi: Different ways. Sometimes I sauté them using olive oil and garlic, or I roast them in the oven. I also like to prepare vegetable purées using abundant onions and green peppers. I'll give you some tips and recipes to cook vegetables when we are done today. Even your children will like them.

Al: Let me tell you, they are not too easy to please.

Emi: Have faith; things may change. Let's make some notes now to wrap up what we have discussed today.

Al's Notes on Salt and Sodium
WHAT I NEED TO DO TO LOWER SODIUM IN MY DIET:

1. When Cooking
   - Either omit salt from recipes or cut the amount in half.
   - Use lemon juice, vinegar, herbs, and spices instead of salt.
   - Add fresh herbs and black pepper to pasta dishes.
   - Use fresh onions, garlic, bell peppers, and tomatoes for sauces.
   - Avoid condiments such as soy sauce or teriyaki sauce.
   - If the recipe calls for tomato sauce or canned vegetables use low sodium or no-salt-added products.
   - Don't add dried soups or bouillon cubes to recipes. They are high in sodium.

- If fresh onions or garlic are not available, use onion or garlic powder. Do not use onion or garlic salt.
- Roast vegetables, such as red peppers and eggplant, to bring out their flavor.

2. At Home
- When buying bread, read the label. It can be high in sodium.
- Include a piece of fruit at all main meals.
- Be careful with breakfast cereals; they can be high in sodium.
- Eat sausage occasionally, but definitely not every day.
- Avoid the salt shaker.
- Stay away from cured foods such as ham, turkey, and bologna.
- Avoid pickles, pickled vegetables, and sauerkraut.
- Avoid condiments such as mustard, ketchup, and barbecue sauce.
- Limit hard cheeses.
- Include a salad at lunch and dinner. Use extra virgin olive oil and lemon or vinegar. Avoid commercial dressings.
- Include two vegetable side dishes with the main entrée.

3. When Eating Out
- Ask the cook or waiter to prepare the food with very little salt or no salt.
- Ask the waiter to take away the salt shaker.
- Have a piece of fruit for dessert.
- Order vegetable side dishes with the main entrée.
- Do not snack on salted nuts; get the raw, unsalted kind.
- Eliminate hot dogs, lunchmeats, sausages, ham, bacon, and any other processed food.

Emi: I'm going to give you a minestrone recipe that will change your mind about vegetables being boring. You can prepare it one of those days when you feel ambitious in the kitchen, then tell me what you think. This dish requires chopping vegetables. Ask your children to help you. Make them part of the process; they may enjoy it.

Al: That will be the day!

Emi: Do you like garlic?

Al: Yes.

Emi: Then, I'm going to give you a recipe for garlic bread. It would be a perfect match for the minestrone.

Al: Thank you very much. I would like to check something with you, if you don't mind.

Emi: Sure, go ahead.

Al: I received a brochure from a local community college offering a Mediterranean cooking class on Saturday mornings. Do you think it may be useful to enroll in the class?

Emi: Absolutely!

Al: The hours are perfect because they don't interfere with my weekly schedule. I'm even tempted to ask my children to enroll with me.

Emi: That's a brilliant idea! Not only will you spend quality time with them, but all of you will learn hands on how to use the ingredients that form part of this wonderful diet. It will be one more step in your journey to recovery and will put your children on the road to prevention, the best cure available.

Al: I'll ask them tonight. The class starts tomorrow and people can register at the door. If they agree, we can all go tomorrow morning.

Emi: Fantastic! Do you have any other questions?

Al: No, that was all. Thank you very much for your advice.

Emi: You're welcome. Monday we'll continue with fruits and vegetables.

Al: Again?

Emi: Yes, but from a different perspective.

REFERENCE

1. Ding EL, Mozaffarian D. Optimal dietary habits for the prevention of stroke. *Seminars in Neurology.* 2006 Feb;26(1):11–23.

Classic Minestrone, Home Version

Makes 4 servings

Ingredients

3 tablespoons olive oil
1 large yellow onion
2 carrots
1 zucchini
4 ounces whole green beans
2 stalks celery
6 cups water
½ cup elbow macaroni
1 14-ounce can chopped tomatoes, no salt added
2 cloves of garlic, crushed
1 teaspoon fresh thyme leaves
　　or ½ teaspoon dried thyme
salt and black pepper
1 14-ounce can kidney beans, low sodium

Preparation

Dice vegetables to ½-inch size. Heat the oil in a pan over medium heat. Add all the fresh vegetables and heat until sizzling. Then cover, lower the heat, and simmer the vegetables for 15 minutes.

Add the water, tomatoes, herbs, and seasoning. Bring to boil, put the lid back, and simmer for about 30 minutes. Add the beans and their liquid together with the pasta and simmer for 10 more minutes until the pasta is tender. Check the seasoning.

Bread With Tomato and Garlic

Makes 4 servings

Ingredients

4 slices fresh bread, whole grain
1 clove of garlic, cut in half
1 ripe tomato
4 tablespoons extra virgin olive oil

Preparation

Cut slices of fresh bread a half-inch thick and toast them. Cut a clove of garlic and rub the bread with it. Then, cut a tomato in half and rub the bread with it. Put a tablespoon of extra virgin olive oil on each slice. It tastes delicious as a snack and is the perfect match for any dish.

Variation

Rub the bread with the garlic. Mix small pieces of fresh tomato, basil, 1 clove of crushed garlic, and extra virgin olive oil. Add the mixture to the bread.

Green Beans With Garlic

Makes 4 to 6 servings

Ingredients

    4 garlic gloves
    1 pound green beans
    extra virgin olive oil
    black pepper

Preparation

Peel 4 or 5 garlic cloves and cut them in small pieces. Crush them in the mortar and leave them there until you have the green beans ready. Once washed, trim the tops and tails from the beans and cut them in half. Steam them for 3 to 5 minutes. Do not overcook; beans should be crisp and bright.

Pour 3 or 4 tablespoons of extra virgin olive oil cold pressed in a frying pan. Heat until the oil is hot. Sauté the garlic stirring it until it starts to brown.

Add the beans to the frying pan, mixing them with the garlic for a couple of minutes. Add the black pepper. Serve warm.

You don't need to add salt. The flavor of the olive oil combined with the garlic is enough to make this healthy dish very tasty. If you still feel you need some salt you can add a pinch to the water you use to steam the beans.

This dish is a great accompaniment to almost any meal.

Variation

Add some diced fresh tomatoes to the frying pan for a half-minute, and you will have a perfect side dish.

Chapter Five

Fruits and Vegetables: Medicine of the Future

Counseling Session—Day 4
Monday, 4:00 P.M.

Emi (*Al enters Emi's office with a grin from ear to ear*): You look happy today. Anything you would like to tell me?

Al: Yes! I went to the cooking class Saturday morning. It was a lot of fun.

Emi: Did your children go with you?

Al: Yes.

Emi: What was their reaction when you asked them to enroll in the class with you?

Al: Well, at first, they didn't like the idea too much because on Saturdays they like to sleep late but finally they agreed to go. When we got to the class, they were a little shy, but soon they got involved in the cooking, and I could tell they were enjoying themselves. By the time we left, they were very happy they came.

Emi: What did you do in the class?

Al: First, the teacher showed us some of the basic ingredients of the Mediterranean diet: extra virgin olive oil, tomatoes, onions, garlic, green peppers, herbs—you know. And then we cooked a couple of Mediterranean dishes.

Emi: What did you prepare?

Al: We made spaghetti sauce and ratatouille (*pisto manchego*). I brought the recipes with me in case you wanted to try them.

Emi: Of course! Thank you very much. So, now you're on your way to becoming a chef.

Al: Well, the children and I left the class so inspired we decided to surprise my wife and do the cooking that night.

Emi: You did? That's fantastic! What did you guys make?

Al: Minestrone. We used the recipe you gave me.

Emi: Was it good?

Al: It was very tasty. We also prepared a fruit salad following your suggestions.

Emi: Which one?

Al: We cut apples and strawberries, and we added some yogurt, raisins, and walnuts. The salad was also very good. I think the fact that the fruit was organic made a difference.

Emi: Yes, as I mentioned, organic fruits are sweeter. Well, you made my day today! This experience will not only help you with your health but at the same time it will help the entire family.

Al: Yes. I was very happy to share these activities with my children because I believe it will help them in the long run. I want my children to live a long life free of disease.

Emi: Absolutely. Making them part of these pastimes will get them familiar with eating healthy foods. And by the way, are you changing your mind about vegetables being boring?

Al: I suppose. Last Friday you said that today we're going to talk about fruits and vegetables, right?

Emi: Yes. Besides the benefits we have seen so far, fruits and vegetables are also indispensable in the fight against heart disease because they have potent *antioxidants*, compounds that prevent or repair the damage caused to our arteries by *free radicals*. This damage, called *oxidation*, is a major culprit in cardiovascular disease.

Al: You mentioned free radicals during our discussions but I don't think I remember what they are.

Free Radicals, a Physics Review

Emi: As you may recall from Physics 101, the nucleus of an *atom* is surrounded by pairs of *electrons*, but at times an atom may lose an electron. This type of atom is called a free radical, or radical, a highly unstable and destructive *molecule* that in the process of trying to get its "pair," attaches itself to another molecule, altering its structure and functionality. The molecule "attacked" becomes a free radical itself, creating a chain reaction of unstable molecules. These unstable molecules subject our cells to continuous damage, *oxidative stress*, that eventually kills the cells. When radicals kill or damage enough cells in an organism, the organism ages and eventually dies. Free radicals are blamed for many illnesses and are heavily implicated in heart disease.

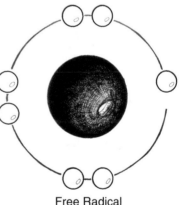

Free Radical

Al: How?

Emi: They can damage the innermost layer of our arteries. I'll explain how this happens.

The Endothelium: The Teflon of Our Arteries

Emi: The inside wall of an artery is protected by a layer of cells called the *endothelium*. A healthy endothelium can be compared to a Teflon coating because it is nonsticky, a quality that allows the blood to flow easily through the arteries. But when the cells of the endothelium are damaged, let's say by free radicals, they fall off from the artery wall leaving that portion of the blood vessel unprotected. This process sets the stage for the formation of plaque in the arteries.

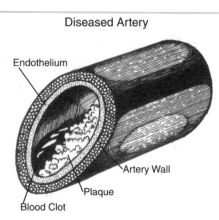

Al: I see. What triggers the formation of free radicals?

Emi: Several things.

What Causes the Formation of Free Radicals?

- Cigarette smoke
- Overexposure to sunlight or smog
- Excessive exercise
- Radiation
- Our own *metabolism* or bodily functions

Emi: All these factors can cause our bodies to become overwhelmed by free radicals, and the natural body mechanisms may not be sufficient to eliminate them.

Al: Why do our bodies form free radicals?

Emi: Some free radicals are formed during normal bodily functions such as eating, drinking, or breathing. Their presence is not always detrimental; for example, free radicals fight viruses and bacteria in our bodies.

Al: Then free radicals are not so bad after all?

Are Free Radicals Bad for Us?

Emi: Free radicals are bad for us when our bodies produce too many. Normally, the body can handle oxidation through special molecules that neutralize radicals before they can damage our cells and cause disease. However, if free radical production becomes excessive or if not enough antioxidants are available, the production of free radicals gets out control.

Al: Then the secret is to keep free radicals at a minimum.

Emi: Exactly!

Al: How do we do that?

How Can We Keep Free Radicals at a Minimum?

Emi: We can keep free radicals at bay by avoiding smoking, over-exposure to sunlight and smog, and excessive exercise. But what is really crucial in the fight against free radicals is to follow a diet abundant in antioxidants.

Al: You said before that antioxidants are molecules that protect our cells, right?

Emi: Yes.

What Are Antioxidants?

Emi: The word *antioxidant* means "against oxidation." The body produces special molecules that fight free radicals. However, when our bodies cannot produce enough of those defense molecules, antioxidants are another kind of compound that helps eliminate free radicals before they can damage our cells and cause diseases. Antioxidants help lower risk of heart attacks by preventing LDL cholesterol oxidation and formation of plaque.

Al: How do antioxidants prevent radical damage?

Emi: By "sacrificing" themselves.

The "Unselfish" Antioxidant

Emi: Antioxidants neutralize radicals by "unselfishly" giving up their own electrons to free radicals. When a free radical gains an electron from an antioxidant, it no longer needs to attack another cell and the chain reaction of oxidation stops there.

Al: But that means the antioxidant becomes a free radical itself, doesn't it?

Emi: Not really. Antioxidants have many protective enzymes and do not become free radicals themselves when they donate an electron. According to Dr. Denham Harman, father of the free radical theory of aging, we can stop reactions before they start or we can decrease the chain of damaging radicals by using antioxidants.

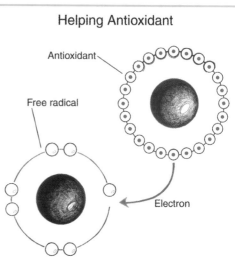

Helping Antioxidant

Antioxidant

Free radical

Electron

Al: If our bodies manufacture antioxidants, why should we worry about free radicals?

Emi: Because there are times when our antioxidant defense system is not strong enough to defend us against those reckless radicals. I'll explain.

Our Antioxidant Defense System

Emi: Although the human body has quite a sophisticated antioxidant defense system to eliminate free radicals, the ability of the cells to produce adequate amounts of antioxidants is determined by factors such as age, genes, nutrition, and stress. In a young and healthy individual, the cells produce sufficient amounts of antioxidants, but as a person grows older, this capacity of the cells is diminished and the antioxidants produced by the body are not enough to face the overproduction of free radicals.

Al: Can we increase the level of antioxidants in our bodies?

Emi: Absolutely.

How Can We Boost Our Antioxidant Defense System?

Emi: We can increase our level of antioxidants by eating plenty of plant foods. Antioxidants such as vitamin E, vitamin C, lycopene, and beta-carotene found in fruits and vegetables supplement the action of our natural body antioxidants, and they can minimize free radical attacks, reducing the risk of many illnesses such as heart disease. The Harvard-based Nurses' Health Studies followed up with about 110,000 men and women for 14 years. The results of the studies showed that compared with the people who ate less than 1.5 servings of fruits and vegetables a day, those who ate 8 or more servings a day were 30 percent less likely to have had a heart attack or stroke. The studies also showed that for every extra serving of fruit and vegetables participants added to their diets, their risk of heart disease dropped by 4 percent.[1] The protective effect of fruits and vegetables was attributed to a category of compounds named *phytochemicals.*

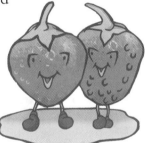

Al: What is that?

Emi: The medicine of the future.

Phytochemicals: Medicine of the Future

Emi: The word "phyto" means "plant" in Greek. Phytochemicals are nonnutritive chemicals found in plant foods that protect their host plants from infections and microbial invasions. Recently, however, we have learned that phytochemicals are also crucial in protecting humans against disease. We know that people who consume plant foods regularly have a lower incidence of heart disease than those who do not include them in their diet. Researchers estimate there are more than 100 different phytochemicals in one serving of fruit or vegetables.

Al: How can phytochemicals protect us?

Phytochemicals Protect Us

Emi: Phytochemicals perform many functions in our bodies. They are involved in the following activities:

- They act as antioxidants.
- They keep the walls of small blood vessels healthy.
- They make our small blood vessels stronger.
- They prevent platelets from becoming sticky and piling up.
- They block specific enzymes that raise blood pressure.

Let's Look at Some of the Main Phytochemicals

CAROTENOIDS

Beta-carotene, lutein, and lycopene

Emi: These protect fat cells, blood, and other body fluids from assault by radicals. They also protect the plants they are part of from the same radicals that attack human cells. Carotenoids are the pigments responsible for the colors of many red, green, yellow, and orange fruits and vegetables. They are found in apricots, cantaloupe, kiwifruit, mangoes, papayas, pink grapefruit, watermelon, broccoli, carrots, kale, pumpkin, spinach, sweet potatoes, winter squash, collard greens, corn, red peppers, romaine lettuce, Swiss chard, and tomatoes. In a few minutes, we'll talk specifically about tomatoes.

FLAVONOIDS

Resveratrol, anthocyanin, quercetin, hesperidin, tangeritin

Emi: Flavonoids are one large family of protective antioxidants commonly seen in foods rich in vitamin C. The activities of flavonoids in our bodies include:

- Acting against inflammation, fighting free radicals, and preventing platelets from sticking together
- Blocking the *enzymes* (proteins that help biochemical reactions to happen) that raise blood pressure
- Protecting and strengthening small blood vessels that carry oxygen and nutrients to all body cells

Al: Wow!

Emi: Because of their antioxidative and antiradical activity, flavonoids are used in pharmaceutical and food industries. According to Kazazic and colleagues, flavonoids have been found to possess significant anti-cardiovascular disease and anti-inflammatory activities.[2]

Al: What foods have flavonoids?

Emi: Flavonoids are found in apples, blueberries, cherries, grapefruit, kiwifruit, limes, oranges, pears, pink grapefruit, plums, red grapes, strawberries, tangerines, broccoli, garlic, kale, lettuce, and onions. Vitamin C is of particular importance in the fight against free radical formation caused by cigarette smoke. Vitamin C also helps return vitamin E to its active form.

Al: What do you mean by that?

Emi: Once vitamin E has been used by our cells, vitamin C comes to the rescue and restores it to its original form, so it can be used again.

Ellagic Acid

Emi: Ellagic acid protects us by decreasing cholesterol levels. It is found in blackberries, blueberries, currants, kiwifruit, raspberries, red grapes, and strawberries. Ellagic is abundant in strawberries and has potent antioxidant power. In studies conducted in labs, strawberry extracts have been shown to inhibit certain enzymes that reduce the inflammation process of arteries.[3]

Allium Compounds

Emi: Allium compounds protect the immune and cardiovascular system. They are found in chives, garlic, leeks, onions, and scallions. The allylic sulfides in these plants are released when the plants are cut or smashed. We'll talk in detail about these compounds when we talk about garlic.

Al: This is really impressive. If antioxidants protect against disease, should I start taking antioxidant supplements?

Emi: That is not advisable.

Al: Why?

Should You Take Antioxidant Supplements?

Emi: Although we know that antioxidants are very helpful in protecting the body against free radical damage, do not rush to the nearest drugstore to stock up on these artificial supplements because we still don't know what their side effects are in the long run. Besides, supplements provide only a few components of the many that occur naturally in fruits and vegetables. Many clinical studies conducted with antioxidant supplements have shown disappointing and frustrating results although we thought them to be "the magic bullet" for preventing hundreds of diseases.[4] Thus, make plant foods your source of antioxidants; they are your best guarantee against disease. Nature provides us with everything we need to enjoy good health; let us take advantage of it.

Al: I understand.

Emi: Let's take a break, and when we come back we'll talk about tomatoes.

Al: Why tomatoes?

Emi: Tomatoes are a must in the fight against heart disease and one of the pillars of the Mediterranean diet.

REFERENCES

1. The Harvard-Based Nurses' Health Study. www.hsph.harvard.edu/nutritionsource/fruits.html.

2. Kazazic SP. Antioxidative and antiradical activity of flavonoids. *Archives of Industrial Hygiene and Toxicology.* 2004 Nov;55(4):279–90.

3. Hannum SM. Potential impact of strawberries on human health: a review of the science. *Critical Reviews in Food Science and Nutrition.* 2004;44(1):1–17.

4. Giugliano D, Esposito K. Mediterranean diet and cardiovascular disease. *Annals of the New York Academy of Sciences.* 2005 Nov;1056:253–60.

Homemade Spaghetti Sauce

Makes 4 servings

Ingredients

extra virgin olive oil
1 large onion, chopped by hand or in a
    food processor
1 green pepper, chopped in small pieces
5 large tomatoes, peeled and cut in small pieces
8 ounces mushrooms, sliced
3 garlic cloves, crushed
thyme, rosemary, oregano
black pepper
pinch of sugar

Preparation

In a frying pan, heat the oil and sauté the onion over low
heat. Before it gets brown add the green pepper. Simmer
until the green pepper is soft. Add the tomatoes. Let it
simmer 8 more minutes. Add the mushrooms. Add the
garlic, thyme, rosemary, oregano, black pepper, and sugar.
Let it cook 10 more minutes. Serve hot over spaghetti.

Pisto Manchego (Ratatouille)

Makes 6 servings

Ingredients

  1 pound zucchini
  ½ pound tomatoes
  6 green peppers
  1 onion, chopped
  extra virgin olive oil
  black pepper

Preparation

You can roast the veggies by arranging them on a lightly oiled wire rack placed over an oven pan, or on a baking sheet covered with lightly oiled foil, in a 450° oven for 15 minutes or until brownish-black specks appear on their surface. Peel the peppers. Mix everything. Sauté in olive oil.

Chapter Six

Tomatoes: A Staple Food for Your Heart

Counseling Session—Day 4 (Continuation)
Monday, after the break

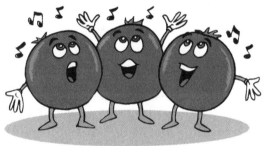

Al: Somebody told me that in the past tomatoes were considered poisonous. How do those stories get started?

Emi: Good question. Europeans were introduced to tomatoes in the 16th century, when the Conquistadors reached Mexico. Despite the tomato's initial acceptance by Southern Europeans, Northerners were hesitant to eat tomatoes because they belong to the same family as the poisonous *nightshade*, a wild plant related to potatoes and eggplants. Thus the British proclaimed the tomato poisonous and stayed away from it. In the meantime, the Mediterranean countries, especially Italy and Spain, welcomed the new fruit, which quickly became a staple to their cuisine.

Al: That explains it! Why are tomatoes so important?

Emi: They are crucial in the fight against heart disease.

Al: Why?

Emi: Because of lycopene.

Al: The term sounds familiar. (*Checking his notes*) Here it is! Now I remember. It's an antioxidant that protects our cells from free radical attacks.

Emi: Exactly.

What Is Lycopene?

Emi: Lycopene is the red pigment found in several fruits and vegetables such as guava, rosehips, watermelon, pink grapefruit, and red chilies, but it mainly comes from tomatoes and tomato products. Recent research has shown that people who eat tomatoes and processed tomatoes on a regular basis are less likely to suffer from heart disease than people who don't eat tomatoes regularly.

Al: Lycopene protects the heart because it fights free radicals, doesn't it?

Emi: Correct. As a powerful antioxidant, lycopene prevents the oxidation of LDL cholesterol caused by radicals. In a study to investigate the effects of tomato lycopene on the oxidation of cholesterol, Agarwal and colleagues provided the participants one-to-two servings per day of tomato juice, spaghetti sauce, and concentrated lycopene for one week. The study showed an important reduction of oxidized LDL cholesterol.[1]

Lycopene can also reduce the amount of cholesterol in the blood. For three months, 60 men were fed 60 milligrams of lycopene per day—the equivalent found in 1 kilo of tomatoes. At the end of the treatment period, the results showed a 14 percent reduction in LDL cholesterol in the blood.[2]

Al: That's an excellent result. I'll stop at the market tonight to buy tomatoes.

Emi: Great! But there is something very important you need to know about tomatoes.

Al: What is that?

Emi: That for lycopene to work in our body, it has to be absorbed by our cells.

Al: What do you mean?

Absorption of Lycopene

Emi: Our tissues have to gulp lycopene from the food we eat and get it inside the cells before they can put it to some use. Research has shown that the level of lycopene found in our organs' tissues is a better indicator of disease prevention than the amount of lycopene we eat.

Al: I see.

Emi: Individuals who have a high concentration of lycopene in their tissues have a lower risk of heart attacks than those who have a low level. In a two-week study conducted by Micozzi, the subjects followed a diet that did not contain lycopene. By the end of the second week, the level of lycopene in the blood of these individuals had decreased by 50 percent and the cholesterol oxidation had increased by 25 percent.[3]

Al: Wow! I definitely need to start eating tomatoes.

Emi: Yes. Research has also shown that lycopene is better absorbed when the meal includes some fat.

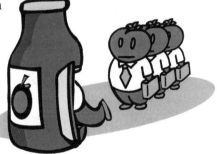

Al: I don't think I follow you now.

Emi: What I'm trying to say is that lycopene appears more readily in the blood if the meal includes a source of fat or if the tomatoes have been heated, as in the case of tomato sauce and tomato paste. Heat changes the chemical structure of lycopene and makes it ready for our cells to swallow it up. Once inside the cells, it is deposited in all our organs. A study published in 1998 showed that our cells absorb lycopene better from processed tomato products than from fresh tomatoes.[4]

Al: What you are saying is that if I eat tomatoes with some kind of fat, I increase the level of absorption and as a result, I also increase the level of antioxidants in my blood?

Emi: Correct.

Al: Does it matter what type of fat I include in the meal?

Emi: No. But the ideal fat is extra virgin olive oil.

Al: What do I have to do to increase the level of lycopene in my body tissues?

Emi: You can do several things.

How to Increase Absorption of Lycopene

- Process the tomatoes with heat. An example would be tomato sauce, tomato paste, or tomato soup.
- Eat fresh tomatoes with fats such as olive oil.
- Eat products that contain lycopene with other food antioxidants.

Al: What do you mean with other antioxidants?

Emi: An example would be eating tomatoes with other vegetables such as in salads or eating a piece of fruit for dessert. Use olive oil and lemon juice as dressing, and you will have the perfect combination of lycopene and antioxidants. In a study conducted by Tyssandier and colleagues, the subjects were supplemented with 96 grams of tomato puree per day for three months. The volunteers then avoided foods rich in tomatoes for the next three weeks. The results showed that including tomato puree in a regular diet significantly increased blood lycopene, beta-carotene, and lutein. Avoiding tomato products for three weeks decreased the level of all antioxidants as well as the total antioxidant capacity of the blood.[5]

Al: You know, this Mediterranean diet sounds quite effective.

Emi: It is. It's based on many ingredients working together as a family that gets on well.

Al: In the past I have tried to make spaghetti sauce but my children didn't like it, so I stopped trying.

Emi: Don't worry. I'll give you a recipe they are sure to like. In the meantime, let's talk about how you can include more tomatoes in your meals.

Ways to Include More Tomatoes in Your Meals

- Make it a point to always have tomatoes at home. Bright red, ripe tomatoes have more lycopene than green or yellow.
- Always include tomatoes in your salads. Use olive oil and lemon or vinegar as dressing.
- Eat pasta with tomato sauce.
- Add some tomato slices to your sandwich.
- Rub half a tomato on the bread you eat with your meal.
- Always keep canned tomatoes—"no salt added"—on hand. They are very handy when you are in a hurry and need them for soups or sauces. One of my favorite brands is Muir Glen Organic— "no salt added," of course.
- Whenever possible, visit your local farmers' market and look for locally grown tomatoes.

Al: How about pizza? Is it a good combination of tomato and fat?

Emi: It's not the ideal combination because the fat is the wrong type, but you can eat pizza in moderation. Ask the waiter or cook to go easy on the cheese and hold the pepperoni and ham.

Al: I read someplace that tomatoes are a fruit? How can a tomato be a fruit?

Emi: Because of vested interests.

Al: What do you mean?

Fruit or Vegetable?

Emi: Botanically speaking, the tomato is a fruit, but from a culinary point of view, it is always grouped with vegetables. In the past, the tomato was classified as a fruit to avoid taxation. But in 1893, the U.S. Supreme Court, using the popular definition that classifies vegetables by their use, settled the controversy by ruling that the tomato was a vegetable and should be taxed accordingly. Based on this popular definition, tomatoes are generally served with dinner and not as dessert.

Al: I guess money talks.

Emi: Yes. Have you ever heard of La Tomatina?

Al: No, what is it?

Emi: A festival.

Tomato Trivia

Emi: Every year, at the peak of the tomato season, the medieval town of Buñol in Valencia, Spain, celebrates a fiesta centered on an enormous tomato fight.

Al: Did you say a "tomato fight"?

Emi: Yes. For two hours, from 11:00 A.M. until 1:00 P.M., the streets of this town turn into rivers of tomato juice as people happily pelt each other with ripe, red tomatoes.

Al: Who started this so-called festival?

Emi: La Tomatina started during the 1940s in Buñol's downtown, when a group of people started a tomato fight.

Al: What triggered the fracas?

Emi: Nobody knows with certainty, but it seems it started as an assault on city officials and extended to some unlucky pedestrians caught in the line of fire.

Al: They must have had a reason for the assault.

Emi: Who knows? Regardless of the motive, it didn't take long for everyone to start having a great time. After this episode, in an effort to draw more tourism (and therefore more targets), the residents of Buñol incorporated La Tomatina as the town's national holiday. Now it has grown into a major fiesta where, for a week, the town is filled with parades, fireworks, food, street parties, and of course, tomatoes.

Al: How fun!

Emi: Yes. The night before La Tomatina, Buñol's narrow streets are filled with more than 100 metric tons of overripe tomatoes waiting impatiently for tens of thousands of visitors from all over the world to participate in this harmless battle.

Al: What a great way to vent stress!

Emi: If you're interested in going, the festival is held on the last Wednesday of August.

Al: I'll check with my wife, and if she agrees I'll call my travel agent. This festival sounds like a good way to get rid of frustrations.

Emi: I agree. Make sure you go dressed to wear tomato juice. Remember you're only allowed to use tomatoes, and you must squish them before slugging them. Any other items are forbidden as they may harm people.

Al: I won't forget.

Emi (*Handing recipe to Al*): I know you have practiced with spaghetti sauce in your Saturday cooking class, but I want to give you a recipe for tomato sauce that you can use with any dish. You can use it with spaghetti, rice, vegetables, or meat.

Al: Thank you very much. (*Looking at the clock on the wall*) I have to run now, I'll see you Wednesday.

REFERENCES

1. Agarwal S, Rao AV. Tomato lycopene and low-density lipoprotein oxidation: a human dietary intervention study. *Lipids.* 1998;33:981–984.

2. Furhman B, Elis A, Aviram M. Hypercholesterolemic effect of lycopene and beta-carotene is related to suppression of cholesterol synthesis and augmentation of LDL receptor activity in macrophage. *Biochemical and Biophysical Research Communications.* 1997;233:658–662 [Medline].

3. Micozzi MS, Brown ED, Edwards BK, et al. Plasma carotenoid response to chronic intake of selected foods and beta-carotene supplements in men. *American Journal of Clinical Nutrition.* 1992;55:1120–1125.

4. Rao AV. Lycopene, tomatoes, and the prevention of coronary heart disease. *Experimental Biology and Medicine.* 2002;227:908–913.

5. Tyssandier V, Feillet-Coudray C, Caris-Veyrat C, et al. Effect of tomato product consumption on the plasma status of antioxidant micro-constituents and on the plasma total antioxidant capacity in healthy subjects. *Journal of the American College of Nutrition.* 2004;23,No. 2,148–156.

Tomato Sauce

Makes 4 servings

Ingredients

2 pounds ripe tomatoes, chopped
2 to 3 tablespoons extra virgin olive oil
thyme
rosemary
oregano
1 bay leaf
black pepper
a pinch of sugar

Preparation

Peel the tomatoes. Heat the oil in a frying pan and add the tomatoes with the rest of the ingredients. Simmer until the water from the tomatoes has evaporated. Adding a pinch of sugar to tomatoes when cooking them enhances the flavor. This sauce can be used with spaghetti, steamed rice, vegetables, or meat.

An easy way to peel fresh tomatoes

Bring a large pot of water to a boil. Drop the tomatoes into the water for 10 to 15 seconds and remove them. Place them in a bowl or sink filled with cold water to cool them down. Cut an "X" through the skin of each tomato and it will easily slip off.

If you are pressed for time, you can use canned tomatoes but you must check the sodium listed on the can. Buy either low sodium (140 milligrams or less) or "no salt added."

Chapter Seven

Is Fat the Villain?

Counseling Session—Day 5
Wednesday, 4:00 P.M.

Emi: Hi, Al. Have a seat, please. I'll be with you in a minute. In the meantime, help yourself to something to drink, please.

Al (*Pulling a can of tomato juice from his brief case*): Thank you, but I brought a can of tomato juice.

Emi: You did?

Al: Yes. After yesterday's discussion, on my way home I stopped at the market and got tomatoes, tomato sauce, and tomato juice.

Emi: Wow! Did you check the sodium in the can?

Al: Yes. This tomato juice is unsalted. It has only 24 milligrams of sodium.

Emi: Excellent! I'm really impressed. Ready to start?

Al: Yes, but first I have to tell you what I did today.

Emi: What did you do?

Al: Yesterday at work, I talked my friend Robert into walking up the stairs with me during our morning break. He's a manager in the receiving department and sometimes we take our breaks at the same time. I didn't know his cholesterol was also high until yesterday, when he confided in me. Anyhow, to make a long story short, I told him what you said about physical activity and he agreed to walk with me. We started today.

Emi: How wonderful! Did you use the whole 15 minutes going up the stairs?

Al: Yes. It took us almost that long to walk up eight floors and come down again.

Emi: Did you get tired?

Al: We stopped on the fourth floor. We rested for a couple of minutes and then continued. Going down was easier. We both felt a sense of accomplishment as we were going down the stairs. It is difficult to explain.

Emi: I know exactly what you mean. I feel the same way every time I come back from my walks. Isn't it a great feeling?

Al: Yes.

Emi: Are you guys going to do this on a regular basis?

Al: Yes. We are going to take our breaks together every day.

Emi: Fantastic! Okay, today we are going to change the subject a little. We are going to explore fats.

Al: You know, this fat business can get quite confusing. Is it true that fat is bad for us?

Emi: Yes and no.

Al (*Looking confused*): What do you mean?

Emi: That not all fats are bad for us. Some fats can be quite harmful, but at the same time we can't survive without fat.

Is Fat Bad for Us?

Emi: Our bodies need fat to function. Among other things, fat provides the *calories* we need to have energy and to be warm; it supplies padding and insulation for our internal organs and maintains healthy skin. Fat transports *vitamins A, D, E, and K* through our blood and helps with their absorption in the intestines. We also need fat to produce *hormones*, chemical substances that control bodily functions.

Al: If fat is so important, why do I keep hearing that it's bad for us?

Emi: Because for the past several decades, and as a result of an epidemic of diseases due to obesity, many organizations have equated healthy eating with a lowfat diet. Consequently, many people have avoided or eliminated foods containing fat from their diets in the belief that they are not good. Scientific research has shown, however, that the type of fat we eat is more important than the amount, and that a lowfat diet that is high in saturated fat would be more harmful to the arteries than a diet high in healthy fats.[1]

Al: That's interesting.

Emi: We also know that people in the Mediterranean countries have fewer heart attacks than people in the United States, although their diets contain higher levels of fat than the diets of the people in this country. Research has shown also that replacing butter and shortening with olive oil lowers the level of cholesterol in the body even if the fat intake remains the same.

Al: Then, why do health authorities keep insisting we follow a diet low in fat?

Emi: Two main reasons:

1. People in Mediterranean countries are physically active throughout their whole lives. Being physically active is a major deterrent to heart disease. Since most people in the United States are on the sedentary side, health authorities fear that encouraging the consumption of foods high in fat could unleash an array of diseases.

2. People in the Mediterranean countries consume mainly olive oil as a source of fat. Olive oil is a healthy fat that does not get stuck in the arteries. On the other hand, people in the United States consume high amounts of *saturated fat* and *trans fats*, two types that can do a lot of harm to our arteries.

Al: Are these two fats the main cause of heart attacks?

Emi: They play a major role in it. When we eat too much saturated fat or trans fats, little by little our arteries can get clogged, preventing the blood from circulating freely. It can cause atherosclerosis.

Al: What foods contain saturated fat?

Emi: Mostly animal fats. Let's walk to the market. It is only a couple of blocks away. I want you to see some food items rich in these two kinds of fat. It will help you identify them in the future. Do you have your notebook with you?

Al: Yes.

Saturated Fat: Villain Number One

Emi (*At the local market*): Let's go to the dairy section. Here, take a look at this butter stick. As you can see, it is solid. Solid fats contain high amounts of saturated fat.

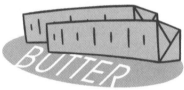

Al: What is the problem with saturated fat?

Emi: Several things:

- Saturated fat is the most rigid of all fats and is solid at room temperature. Solid fats are hard to dissolve and can easily get stuck in our arteries.

- Saturated fat causes the liver to overproduce cholesterol. The liver makes about 75 percent of the cholesterol our body needs from internal sources, while the remaining 25 percent comes from food. But when we eat too much saturated fat, our liver keeps producing cholesterol and we end up with much more cholesterol than we need.

Al: I should not eat anything that has saturated fat?

Emi: As a preventive measure, we should limit saturated fat consumption to less than 10 percent of the total calories ingested per day. In your case, limit it to 7 percent since your blood cholesterol is already high. Unfortunately, in the United States, saturated fat represents between 15 and 20 percent of calories consumed.

Al: How do I know if I am going over the limit?

Emi: Read food labels. Let's look at this label again. Here you can see that the amount of saturated fat is 6 grams. This is awfully close to the recommended daily allowance, so it tells you that this product is not a wise choice.

Al: I see.

Emi: In the dairy section you can find other items containing saturated fat: whole milk, cheese, sour cream, whole yogurt, and many more. When doing the shopping in this section, choose items carefully and always read the labels. Labels are a tremendous source of information and can guide you in choosing food items.

Al: I am pretty sure we buy whole milk at home.

Emi: Talk to your wife. If she happens to be the one going to the market, ask her to buy only 1 percent milk.

Al: Do only dairy products contain saturated fat?

Emi: No. All animal products contain this kind of fat, although in different degrees. Certain plants, such as coconut and palm, are also rich in saturated fat. Let's go now to the meat section.

Nutrition Facts

Serving Size 1 Package (227g)

Amount Per Serving

Calories 270	Calories from Fat 140

	% Daily Value*
Total Fat 16g	24%
Saturated Fat 6g	32%
Cholesterol 55mg	19%
Sodium 1380mg	57%
Total Carbohydrate 20g	7%
Dietary Fiber 2g	7%
Sugars 3g	
Protein 11g	

Vitamin A 8%	•	Vitamin C 8%
Calcium 6%	•	Iron 8%

*Percent Daily Values are based on a 2,000 calorie diet. Your daily values may be higher or lower depending on your calorie needs:

	Calories:	2,000	2,500
Total Fat	Less than	65g	80g
Saturated Fat	Less than	20g	25g
Cholesterol	Less than	300mg	300mg
Sodium	Less than	2,400mg	2,400mg
Total Carbohydrate		300g	375g
Dietary Fiber		25g	30g

Calories per gram:
Fat 9 • Carbohydrate 4 • Protein 4

At the Meat Section

Emi: You need to be selective and read labels when you buy red meat since not all meat cuts are equal. For example, cuts of meat from the ribs and loin areas are the fattiest because the muscles in those areas are not heavily used. Next time you buy meat, use the guidelines outlined in this table.

TABLE #6—FAT CONTENT IN MEAT

3 Grams of Fat per Ounce

Beef	Round, sirloin, and flank steak; tenderloin; roast (rib, chuck, rump); steak (T-bone, porterhouse, cubed); ground round
Pork	Fresh ham; canned, cured, or boiled ham; Canadian bacon; tenderloin; center loin chop
Lamb	Roast, chop or leg
Veal	Lean chop; roast
Chicken, turkey	White meat, no skin

5 Grams of Fat per Ounce

Beef	Most beef products fall into this category (ground beef, meatloaf, corned beef, short ribs, and prime grades of meat trimmed of fat)
Pork	Top loin, chop; Boston butt, cutlet
Lamb	Rib roast, ground
Veal	Cutlet, ground or cubed
Chicken, turkey	Dark meat, no skin

8 Grams of Fat per Ounce

Pork	Spareribs; ground pork; pork sausage
Other	Processed sandwich meats such as bologna, salami, sausages
Chicken, turkey	Dark meat with skin; ground turkey; ground chicken fried chicken with skin

Table #6—Based on the American Dietetic Association and American Diabetes Association guidelines for Exchange Lists for Meal Planning.

Al: This means I don't need to stop eating red meat, right?

Emi: Right. Scientists from Zhejiang University in China reviewed 54 studies conducted on red meat consumption and cardiovascular disease. The studies showed that lean red meat trimmed of visible fat does not raise cholesterol in our blood. In addition, lean red meat is a good source of protein, vitamin B12, zinc, and iron.[2]

Al: I'm glad to hear this because I like red meat.

Emi: Try not to eat it more than a couple of times per week. Buy only the leanest cuts and trim all the outside fat before cooking.

Al: I'll tell my wife.

Emi: When dealing with poultry, choose white meat and remove the skin. You can also follow the guidelines outlined in table 6. As you can see, you can also buy chicken breasts that have the skin already removed.

Al (*Scribbling a few notes and looking at table 6*): There is a big difference in the amount of fat contained in poultry with skin, compared to the one without skin.

Emi: Yes. And remember we are still talking about saturated fat—one of the riskiest when it comes to raising cholesterol in our blood. Now let's go to the oil section where we can find some good fats. They are classified as *monounsaturated* and *polyunsaturated fats*.

Al: What makes them good fats?

Emi: They don't get stuck in our arteries. They also have many other benefits.

Monounsaturated Fats Protect Our Hearts

Emi: Most monounsaturated fats are liquid at room temperature. These kinds of fats protect our hearts because they:

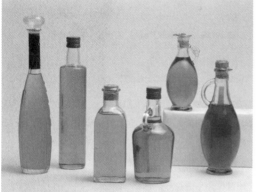

Various bottles of olive oil.
Photo by J.A. Sanguinetti. Courtesy of Diputación Provincial de Jaen, Spain.

- Don't get stuck in our arteries since they are liquid and flow through our blood vessels.
- Lower LDL, the bad cholesterol.
- Don't lower HDL, the good cholesterol; some may even raise it.
- Are not converted into cholesterol as happens with saturated fat.

As you can see, this type of fat contributes to a healthy heart. Populations with diets high in monounsaturated fats, such as those in Mediterranean countries where olive oil is commonly used, have a mortality rate from heart disease that is half that of the United States. Studies have shown that replacing saturated fat with monounsaturated fat reduces the bad cholesterol and increases the good.

Al: What products contain monounsaturated fat?

Emi: The main sources are olive and canola oil. We'll talk in depth about olive oil next week. Nuts are also rich in monounsaturated fats. Participants in one group in the European study PREDIMED were treated with nuts. This group obtained the same beneficial effects—lower cholesterol and lower blood pressure—as the group consuming olive oil.

Al: How many nuts did they have to eat per day to obtain those results?

Emi: The amount of nuts provided daily to the group was:
- 15 grams walnuts (about 3 units)
- 7.5 grams almonds (about 6 units)
- 7.5 grams hazelnuts (about 8 units)

Al: I like nuts. Can I have nuts as a snack?

Emi: Certainly. Try to stay close to the amount set by the study. To reap the health benefits of nuts, buy them raw and keep them in the refrigerator to prevent them from getting rancid. You can have them either for breakfast or as a snack during the day. Another healthy fat that should be part of your diet is polyunsaturated fat, although this type of fat has a catch and should be eaten in moderation.

Al: What do you mean?

Polyunsaturated Fats

Emi: Polyunsaturated fats don't get stuck in our arteries, but because of their chemical structure, they are a favorite target of free radicals. When fats are "attacked" by free radicals, the fat cells become oxidized. We have already seen that oxidation can cause cells to malfunction and die. Polyunsaturated fats should be limited to a certain degree because, although they lower LDL, the "bad" cholesterol, they also lower HDL cholesterol, the "good" one.

Al: What are the sources of polyunsaturated fats?

Emi: Sources include corn, safflower, sunflower, and soybean oils. Mediterraneans don't consume these oils too often, which could contribute to the lower incidence of heart disease among them.

Al: How about fish? Can I eat fish?

Emi: Absolutely! Do you like it?

Al: Yes.

Emi: Let's head over to the fish section.

Fish and Omega-3 Oils

Emi: Fish, especially "oily fish," should be part of your diet. It is high in two main *omega-3 oils* (fatty acids)—EPA and DHA.

Al: What are omega-3 oils?

Emi: Omega-3 oils are a type of polyunsaturated fat that our body needs but cannot manufacture or can only manufacture in insufficient amounts. Without these oils the body cannot perform certain vital functions, thus, we need to get it from the foods we eat. We know through studies that omega-3 oils reduce the risk for heart attacks and strokes.

Al: How?

Emi: Research has shown that they:

- Decrease risk of *arrhythmias*, which can lead to sudden cardiac death.
- Decrease triglyceride levels. This is an area where omega-3 oils have proved to be quite effective.
- Reduce the formation of clots. A major effect of omega-3 oils is reducing the stickiness of platelets in the blood thus decreasing the risk for blockage of the arteries.
- Reduce inflammation of blood vessels.
- Dilate the blood vessels, keeping blood flowing smoothly, which helps lower blood pressure.

Al: What fish are considered oily?

Emi: Mainly salmon, sardines, tuna, and mackerel.

Al: How much fish should I eat?

Emi: The American Heart Association recommends consuming two fish meals per week. Individuals at risk for heart disease benefit from the consumption of higher intakes of fish high in omega-3 oils, although the ideal intake is not clear yet.[3] A study conducted by Harvard University showed that women who ate fish more than once a month had a lower risk of heart attacks than women who only ate fish once a month.[4]

Al: I heard I shouldn't eat fish because it is contaminated from substances found in the waters, such as mercury.

Emi: Yes, but the levels of contamination are generally higher in older and larger fish.

Al: How does mercury get into the water?

Emi: Most mercury pollution comes from manufacturing plants. The burning of coal releases mercury into the air. The mercury enters the water cycle when it rains and then it moves into the bodies of large carnivorous fish such as swordfish and mackerel. Big fish eat small- and medium-sized fish, so they end up with much more mercury in their bodies. Buy small fish to minimize this problem.

Al (*Looking at his notes*): At the beginning of our discussion you mentioned trans fats. What are they?

Emi: Trans fats are the worst of all fats. Come with me.

Hydrogenated Oils or Trans Fats: Villain Number Two

Emi (*Walking along the market aisles*): *Hydrogenated oils*, or trans fats as they are usually called, are produced artificially by inserting molecules of hydrogen in vegetable oils, a process called *hydrogenation*. Through this process, the oil, which is liquid at room temperature, changes its original form and becomes solid. In other words, it becomes a saturated fat.

Al: Why on earth do manufacturers do that?

Emi: Several reasons. Products containing trans fats can stay fresh longer, which means an improved shelf life. Food markets can keep products containing hydrogenated oils on the shelves for years without becoming stale. In addition, they are inexpensive.

Al: Well, based on what you're telling me, they sound like a great invention.

Emi: They are for the manufacturers, but not for our hearts. Health authorities are concerned that the consumption of trans fats might have contributed to the 20th century epidemic of coronary heart disease because they are compounds that have unnatural shapes.

Al: What do you mean by unnatural shapes?

Emi: Because of the process of hydrogenation, the original fat ends up with a different chemical structure that can harm our body organs.

Al: How do compounds with unnatural shapes cause damage in our bodies?

Emi: The unnatural shapes of trans fats cause our cells to become malformed and to malfunction. And that includes the cells of the heart and arteries.

Al: Good God! What kinds of foods have trans fats?

Foods That Contain Trans Fats

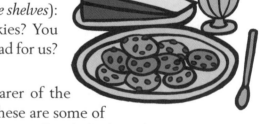

Emi (*Stopping at the cookie aisle*): These are some of the products containing trans fats.

Al (*Looking at the cookie shelves*): Which ones? Cookies? You mean, cookies are bad for us? Why?

Emi: Sorry to be the bearer of the bad news but yes, these are some of the items that have trans fats: baked goods containing high amounts of fat such as croissants, cookies, cakes, donuts, and the like.

Al: How terrible! And here I was eating a croissant every day! I have already replaced the croissant with whole grain bread as you suggested but this means I won't be able to eat cookies or cake ever again!

Emi: That's not true. Of course, you cannot eat commercial baked goods every day if you want to take care of your heart and arteries, but you can have them occasionally. Here is an idea. Tonight, when you get home, make a list of all your relatives' and closest friends' birthdays. Throw one party every month to celebrate their birthday anniversaries. This will give you an excuse to eat cake and cookies, and your friends and family will love you.

Al (*Al goes back to his notebook with a frown and makes a few notes*): That might be too expensive. Eating trans fats affects my cholesterol?

Emi: Yes.

Al: How?

Consequences of Eating Foods Containing Trans Fats

Emi: Trans fats can hurt us because they:

- Raise LDL cholesterol, the "bad" guy. Through the manufacturing process, a liquid oil becomes saturated. We have already seen that the liver uses saturated fat to produce more cholesterol than we need.
- Lower HDL cholesterol, the "good" guy.
- Damage the arteries, setting the stage for the formation of plaque. Plaque clogs the arteries.

Al: I guess they are not such a great invention after all.

Emi: As I said before, not for the consumer.

Al: Any other foods that have trans fats?

Emi: Yes, 50 percent of trans fats come from animal foods that are high in fat. The other 50 percent come from hydrogenated vegetable oils. Examples of foods containing trans fats include:

- Animal foods high in fat—beef, butter, and milk fats
- Snack foods such as crackers and potato chips
- Stick margarine and shortening
- Baked goods high in fat, such as cookies, cakes, croissants, and the like
- Fried foods in fast food restaurants

Scientific evidence showing that trans fats may have contributed to the epidemic of heart disease is so overwhelming, the Food and Drug Administration had to issue a proposal to include the content of trans fats on food labels. As a result, starting January 2006, manufacturers of packaged foods have to disclose the amount of trans fats per serving contained in the package. Restaurants have already or are currently working on outlawing the use of trans fats. When eating out, whether at a restaurant, a bakery, or any other place, ask if they use partially hydrogenated oil for frying or baking. Unless you know otherwise, always assume that almost all labeled baked and fried goods contain hydrogenated oil.

Al: Thank you for such wonderful advice. I though margarine was good for people because it has no cholesterol.

Emi: In the past we assumed that margarine was better for the heart because it's produced from vegetable oils and has no cholesterol; however, it's made from hydrogenated oils and contains large amounts of trans fats. If you ever use margarine, use the liquid type. Of course, replacing margarine and butter with olive oil is still a better strategy to prevent heart disease.

Al: I see. The food label will tell me if the product has trans fats?

Emi: Most of the time. Food manufacturers do not have to list the amount of trans fats if the total fat in the food is less than 0.5 grams per serving.

Al: That means I still may be eating trans fats and not be aware of it.

Emi: If hydrogenated oil is one of the ingredients in the product, then it has trans fats, although in small amounts. Read the label and look for the words "trans fats" and "hydrogenated oil." The report issued by the Institute of Medicine in 2002 doesn't set maximum levels for trans fats but any amount above zero is a risk. Therefore, the report recommendation is to eat as little trans fats as possible while consuming a diet adequate in other important nutrients.[5] Eat lowfat dairy products and lowfat meats, and for dessert, replace commercial baked goods with fruit. These steps will go a long way in helping you reduce the amount of trans fats in your diet. Let's go back to my office. We need to talk about cholesterol.

REFERENCES

1. Hu F, Meir J. Stampfer M, Manson J, Rimm E, Graham A, Colditz G, Rosner B, Hennekens CH, Willett W. Dietary fat intake and the risk of coronary heart disease in women. *New England Journal of Medicine.* 1997 Nov 20;Vol 337:1491–1499, No. 21.

2. Li D, Siriamornpun S, Wahlqvist M, Mann N, Sinclair A. Lean meat and heart health. Department of Food Science and Nutrition, Zhejiang University. *Asia Pacific Journal of Clinical Nutrition.* 2005;14(2):113–9.

3. Kris-Etherton P, Harris W, Appel L. Fish consumption, fish oil, omega-3 fatty acids, and cardiovascular disease. *Circulation.* 2002;106:2747.

4. Hu, F, Willett W, Stampfer M, Rexrode K, Albert C, Hunter D, Manson J. Fish and omega-3 fatty acid intake and risk of coronary heart disease in women. Department of Nutrition, Harvard School of Public Health, *Journal of the American Medical Association.* 2002 Apr 10;287(14):1815–21.

5. Institute of Medicine. Dietary reference intakes for energy, carbohydrate, fiber, fat, fatty acids, cholesterol, protein, and amino acids. Washington, DC: National Academies Press, 2002.

Chapter Eight

If It Has a Mother and a Father, It Has Cholesterol

Counseling Session—Day 5 (Continuation)
Wednesday. back at the office

Al: Is cholesterol a fat?

Emi: Not exactly.

Al: What is it?

What Is Cholesterol?

Emi: Cholesterol is a waxy substance made by the liver that looks like fat but has a different chemical structure. Despite the bad press it has earned over the years because of its involvement in heart disease, cholesterol is vital for our health; it's necessary to build our cell walls and to perform other important functions such as manufacturing hormones, vitamin D, and *bile acids*, the acids our bodies need to help digest food. When the cholesterol level jumps above normal, however, it becomes a risk factor for heart disease.

Al: Why?

Emi: Because too much cholesterol can lead to *atherosclerosis*, the clogging of the arteries.

Al: How do we end up with too much cholesterol in our system?

Emi: Several ways. Let me explain.

How Do We Get High Cholesterol?

1. We are not physically active. Physical activity lowers the cholesterol in our blood.
2. Our diet is too high in animal products. Cholesterol is found in red meat, poultry, fish, eggs, and dairy products.
3. Our liver makes more cholesterol than our body needs when we eat too much saturated fat or trans fats.
4. Our liver manufactures too much cholesterol because we inherited the wrong genes from our parents.

Al: If I have the wrong genes, there is nothing I can do about my high cholesterol?

Emi: Yes, you can. It's true that you cannot change your genes—it's too late to change your parents by now—but if you are physically active and follow certain dietary guidelines, you can go a long way in keeping your cholesterol level under control.

Al: Do fruits and vegetables have cholesterol?

Emi: No. Only foods that have a mother and a father have cholesterol.

Al: Ah! I didn't know that.

Emi: The liver is the organ in charge of manufacturing cholesterol; since plants don't have a liver, they don't have cholesterol either. Let's take a look at some of the different types of cholesterol we have in our bodies.

Total Cholesterol

Emi: Total cholesterol is the sum of the different types of cholesterol found in the blood. Cholesterol levels are measured in milligrams (mg) of cholesterol per deciliter (dl) of blood.

Al: Is my total cholesterol level too high?

Emi (*Reaching for a cholesterol table*): This table shows the guidelines established by the National Cholesterol Education Program. Take a look and compare it with your cholesterol values.

TABLE #7—TOTAL CHOLESTEROL

Total Cholesterol (milligrams per deciliter)	
Desirable	Less than 200 mg/dl
Borderline high	200 to 239 mg/dl
High	240 mg/dl or higher

Table #7—The National Cholesterol Education Program.

Al: Oh my! My total cholesterol is 240 milligrams per deciliter. Based on this table, I am at the top. This is serious, isn't it?

Emi: Yes, because the higher your total cholesterol level is, the higher your chance of developing heart disease. The Multiple Risk Factor Intervention Trial study evaluated 356,222 men for seven years. The researchers found that men with total cholesterol above 220 milligrams per deciliter had twice the risk of dying of heart disease than men with total cholesterol of 180 milligrams per deciliter or less. Men with readings of 245 milligrams per deciliter tripled the risk. It was estimated that 46 percent of the deaths due to heart disease were attributable to blood cholesterol levels of 180 milligrams per deciliter or greater.[1]

Al: This is horrible! Am I going to die?

Emi: None of us lives forever, but you still have time to change your lifestyle and see an improvement in your lab tests. Let's take a look at the other types of cholesterol.

Types of Cholesterol

Emi: Although there are several classifications of cholesterol, the two main ones are LDL cholesterol or *low-density lipoproteins*, known as "bad" cholesterol and HDL cholesterol, or *high-density lipoproteins*, known as "good" cholesterol.

Al: What are *lipoproteins?*

Emi: They are a combination of protein and fat (lipo is another word for fat). Lipoproteins can be compared to transportation vehicles, sort of like buses.

Al: That's interesting! Why?

Emi: Cholesterol has to move from the liver to our cells so it can do its job—build and repair cell walls and manufacture certain body compounds. Because cholesterol is a fatty substance and cannot navigate in watery blood, it goes from place to place in special vehicles called *lipoproteins*. The outside of these "buses" is made of protein, and the cholesterol, the "passenger," travels comfortably inside. Lipoproteins deliver cholesterol to the cells and pick up the cholesterol the cells don't need to be shuttled out of the body.

Al: How fascinating!

Emi: Let's see how LDL cholesterol, the "bad" guy, works.

LDL Cholesterol, the "Bad" Guy

Emi: Low-density lipoproteins are just one type of "bus" that navigates in our blood carrying cholesterol from the liver to our organs. After the cells have taken the amount of cholesterol they need to perform their tasks, the "buses" dump the remaining LDL cholesterol in our blood vessels. As you can imagine, this causes major problems because loose cholesterol in our blood gets deposited in the artery walls and forms plaque. When plaque forms in the arteries that supply blood to the heart, it can cause heart attacks. This is the reason why LDL is known as the "bad" cholesterol.

Al: Are total cholesterol and LDL levels the same?

Emi: No, they are different. Here is the table with the LDL cholesterol values.

TABLE #8—LDL CHOLESTEROL

LDL Cholesterol (milligrams per deciliter)	
Optimal	Less than 100 mg/dl
Near optimal	100 to 129 mg/dl
Borderline high	130 to 159 mg/dl
High	160 to 189 mg/dl
Very high	190 mg/dl and above

Table #8—The National Cholesterol Education Program.

Al: Let me check mine. This is pathetic! My LDL is 150.

Emi: Yes, but it will go down. Keep up the good work, and you will see different results on your next visit to the lab.

HDL Cholesterol, the "Good" Guy

Emi: The other major kind of lipoprotein is high-density lipoprotein or HDL cholesterol, the "good" one. High density lipoproteins are also part of the "bus transportation system," but the role of these "buses" is the opposite of LDL cholesterol. They remove excess cholesterol from our arteries and transport it to the liver, which breaks it down for excretion. Because this type of lipoprotein prevents the accumulation of cholesterol in the blood and is associated with a lower risk of heart disease, it is known as "good" cholesterol. Research has shown that high levels of HDL are the best guarantee of survival in people who have undergone heart surgery. Table #9 lists the guidelines for HDL cholesterol levels.

TABLE #9—HDL CHOLESTEROL

HDL Cholesterol (milligrams per deciliter)

Desirable	60 mg/dl or higher HDL levels of 60 mg/dl or more help lower the risk of heart disease
Low	Less than 40 mg/dl Less than 40 mg/dl is considered a major risk factor for heart disease

Table #9—The National Cholesterol Education Program.

Al: Well, at least my HDL is not as outrageously bad as the other two.

Emi: Right. Your HDL is 43 milligrams per deciliter, but we need to work on improving it.

Al: How about my triglycerides? Are they high?

Emi: Let's look.

TABLE #10—TRIGLYCERIDES

Triglycerides (milligrams per deciliter)

Normal	Less than 150 mg/dl
Borderline high	150 to 199 mg/dl
High	200 to 499 mg/dl
Very high	500 mg/dl or higher

Table #10—The National Cholesterol Education Program.

Al: Not doing too well in this department either! Exactly how does cholesterol block the arteries?

Emi: Cholesterol can hurt us when it gets damaged by free radicals (oxidation).

Al: You've lost me here.

Emi: If you remember from our discussion of free radicals and antioxidants, when the endothelium, the tissue that covers the inside of the arteries, is damaged, plaque can form. The major factor that triggers the formation of this plaque is damaged or oxidized cholesterol.

Al: Is that bad?

Emi: Very.

Damage (Oxidation) of LDL Cholesterol Inside the Arteries

Emi: LDL cholesterol navigating through our arteries is protected against oxidation because the blood contains a fair amount of antioxidants. However, artery walls do not have such a protection, and when LDL cholesterol penetrates them, as happens when the endothelium is damaged, the molecules of cholesterol are "attacked" by the free radicals produced by artery walls. This process damages the cholesterol. When cholesterol is oxidized, it can alter coagulation patterns in the blood, causing the formation of *platelets*, which in turn leads to the formation of plaque. Plaque causes the narrowing of the arteries, interfering with the normal blood flow in the blood vessels. Eventually the blood vessel may be shut down completely, causing a heart attack or a stroke.

Al: What a nightmare! How can we prevent this process?

Emi: By preventing cholesterol from getting oxidized.

Al: How can we do that?

Emi: By doing the following:
- Being physically active.
- Minimizing the amount of saturated fat in the diet.
- Following the guidelines recommended by health authorities for cholesterol consumption.

- Eating abundant plant foods. Plant foods are the ones that can help us with this oxidation business because they take apart free radicals.

Al: What are some of the foods I can eat that contain "good" cholesterol?

Emi: None.

Do Foods Have "Good" or "Bad" Cholesterol?

Emi: Foods don't have good or bad cholesterol; it is all the same. "Good" and "bad" cholesterol refers to the proportion of cholesterol compared to the proportion of proteins that form the lipoproteins, not the type of cholesterol. If the lipoprotein has more cholesterol than protein, we call it "bad" cholesterol. If the lipoprotein has more protein than cholesterol, we call it "good" cholesterol.

Al: Is there a limit on the amount of cholesterol I can eat?

Emi: Yes.

How Much Cholesterol Can You Eat?

Emi: Nutrition experts recommend limiting cholesterol intake to 300 milligrams per day. But keep in mind that although you need to watch for cholesterol in your diet, a major source of cholesterol comes from saturated fat and trans fats. Thus, when you think about decreasing cholesterol from food, don't forget that the real villains are saturated fat and trans fats.

Al: How can I lower my "bad" cholesterol and increase the "good" one?

Emi: You need to do the following:

- Be physically active; this is an ingredient that for centuries has protected those in Mediterranean countries from high cholesterol, high blood pressure, and consequently, heart attacks.
- Keep saturated fat and trans fats at a minimum.

- Keep cholesterol intake at 300 milligrams or lower.
- Replace bad fats with healthy fats such as olive oil.

Al: I'm telling you, my hair stands on end when dealing with fats!

Emi: Don't worry. The goal of our discussions is to get you familiar with which foods you need to emphasize and which you need to avoid or minimize. Let's review some steps you can take to reduce harmful fats in your diet while including more healthy fats.

Al Makes the Following Notes:
AT THE SUPERMARKET

- *Red meat.* Choose only very lean cuts. Buy meat at stores such as Whole Foods. The cattle sold in this type of store are left to graze in open fields, thus the meat is not so fatty.
- *Poultry.* Choose white meat. When possible, buy free range chickens; their meat has less fat because they are left loose to obtain food instead of being caged, and with exercise they develop more muscle and less fat.
- *Cheese.* Choose one that is low in fat. One ounce of hard cheese may range from 3 to 5 grams of saturated fat. One ounce of cheese is about the size of a 1-inch cube.
- *Milk.* Choose 1 percent milk. Two percent milk still contains a lot of saturated fat.
- *Yogurt.* Choose nonfat yogurt. Lowfat yogurt is still high in saturated fat.
- *Processed foods.* Keep these foods at a minimum. Read the labels to identify saturated fats and trans fats.
- *High fat baked goods.* Croissants, donuts, cookies, and cakes are very high in saturated fat and trans fats. They are the foundation for high cholesterol.
- *Snack foods.* Avoid crackers, potato chips, and products that are made with partially hydrogenated oils; they are a main source of *trans* fats.

- *Margarine.* Stick margarine is made with partially hydrogenated oil and contains trans fats. Buy the liquid form.
- *Vegetable shortening.* It is made with hydrogenated oil, the source of trans fats.
- *Cold cuts.* Meats such as ham, turkey, bologna, and salami are very high in saturated fat. Also be wary of sausage, which is high in fat. Eat these items sparingly.

AT HOME

- *Baked products high in fat.* Replace croissants or donuts with whole wheat or whole grain breads.
- *Fruit.* Include a piece of fruit or a fruit salad in your meals. Make a piece of fruit your dessert.
- *Eggs.* Limit scrambled eggs to three times a week. Make them with one whole egg and two whites instead of with two whole eggs. Eggs are a good source of protein, but the yolk is high in cholesterol and should not be eaten every day.
- *Meat.* Trim all the outside fat before cooking and when served to minimize the amount of saturated fat. Limit intake of meat to two servings or less per day. One serving is 3 ounces of cooked meat (4 ounces uncooked). Most meats contain a similar amount of cholesterol, about 70 milligrams in each 3-ounce cooked serving (about the size of a deck of cards).
- *Chicken.* Select white meat and take the skin off.
- *Vegetables.* Sautée vegetables with extra virgin olive oil instead of butter. This oil does not get stuck in the arteries.
- *Cheese and butter.* Don't eat butter and cheese every day.
- *Dry beans.* Include dry beans, lentils, and garbanzo beans in the menu as a main entrée. Legumes, when combined with grains such as bread or rice, provide high quality protein and as we'll see, they lower cholesterol.
- *Salad dressings.* Stay away from commercial salad dressings. Use extra virgin olive oil and lemon or vinegar as dressing.

AT RESTAURANTS

- *Salads.* Choose a salad or prepare one from the salad bar. Use olive oil and lemon or vinegar as dressing. Commercial dressings have a lot of saturated fat. Be wary of lowfat dressings. They may be loaded with trans fats. Ask the server if the dressing is made with partially hydrogenated oil.
- *Soup.* Choose vegetable, chicken, or legume soups such as lentils or dry beans. They are much lower in saturated fat than cream soups, which are usually made with whole milk products.
- *Chicken.* Best choice is white meat, grilled.
- *Fish.* When available, choose fish as the main entrée. Fish contains omega-3 oils, which are good for the heart. Best choice is grilled.
- *Vegetables.* Order vegetables as side dishes.
- *Fruit.* Eat a piece of fruit for dessert, rather than cookies or cake.
- *Sauces.* Stay away from dishes made with heavy sauces because most of the time they are made with whole cream, which means saturated fat.
- *Pasta.* When having pasta, choose a dish made with tomato sauce, garlic, and olive oil. It is an excellent dish for a healthy heart.
- *Deep-fried foods.* Avoid these foods. Many restaurants use partially hydrogenated oils in their fryers, which translates into trans fats.

Al: Do I need to stop eating ice cream?

Emi: You can have some on your birthday.

Al: I was afraid you would say that.

Emi: I hate to be a party pooper but to make up for it, I'll give you a couple of fish recipes since I know you like it.

Al (*Looking discouraged*): Okay.

Emi: Do you have any questions about your notes?

Al: I do. I don't know how on earth Jane, the woman in charge of writing the company's newsletter, learned that I'm attending a Mediterranean cooking class, but she asked me to contribute a recipe to the newsletter. Do you mind if I give her the minestrone and garlic bread recipes you gave me?

Emi: Not at all! The idea is to spread the word so other people can benefit.

Al: Thank you very much. I'll talk to Jane tomorrow. I'm sure she'll be very happy.

REFERENCE

1. Stamler J, Wentworth D, Neaton JD. Prevalence and prognostic significance of hypercholesterolemia in men with hypertension. Prospective data on the primary screenees of the Multiple Risk Factor Intervention Trial. *American Journal of Medicine.* 1986 Feb 14;80(2A):33–9.

Potatoes With Fish

Makes 4 servings

Ingredients

½ pound green peas
olive oil
2 onions
2 cloves of garlic
2 pounds potatoes
salt
black pepper
3 tablespoons fresh parsley, chopped
1 pound of fish, skinned and boneless (try hake,
    sea bass, cod, or haddock)

Preparation

Cook the green peas in a steamer and set aside. In a frying pan, heat the oil and sauté the onions for 5 minutes. Add the garlic and potatoes. Cover with water and season. When the potatoes are tender add the parsley, green peas, and fish. Let it cook a little longer until ready. Serve hot.

Hake With Tomato Sauce

Makes 4 servings

Ingredients

2 pounds hake
salt
bread crumbs
4 tablespoons extra virgin olive oil
1 onion
2 green peppers, chopped
1 16-ounce can tomato sauce, low sodium
3 cloves of garlic, crushed
parsley
black pepper

Preparation

Sprinkle the hake with salt and roll it in the bread crumbs. In a frying pan heat the oil and sauté the onion and green peppers. Add the tomato sauce, parsley, and black pepper and let it simmer for 5 more minutes. Pour the sauce over the hake and bake until done (30 to 45 minutes). Add the garlic last.

Chapter Nine

Olive Oil: "Liquid Gold"

Counseling Session—Day 6
Friday, 4:00 P.M., Emi's office

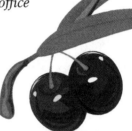

Al: I gave Jane the recipes. She liked them very much. She is giving me credit in the newsletter.

Emi: You are on your way to becoming a celebrity in your company.

Al: Actually, Jane wants to start a health column in the newsletter and has asked me if I want to collaborate with her. That would mean writing a small article every month and providing her with recipes. I told her I'll get back to her.

Emi: You can give her some of the recipes I'm giving you and some of those you are getting from your Mediterranean cuisine class.

Al: Yeah, I suppose I can do that. I'll tell Jane I'll contribute some of my "expertise" to the newsletter. I like the idea of other people benefiting from healthy cooking. (*Looking at several bottles of olive oil*) I remember you saying that today we are going to look at olive oil. Is it true it is good for our health? Lately I hear a lot of people talking about this oil.

Emi: Very good! For centuries olive oil has been a major player in the low incidence of heart disease among Mediterranean populations. Although the health and longevity of the Mediterranean people are associated with a diet high in plant foods and low in animal products, what has really defined this traditional diet is the abundant use of olives and olive oil, the principal fat source and the culinary foundation of the Mediterranean cuisine.

Al: I eat olives once in a while with my meals.

Emi: They are good for you but olives can be high in sodium. Read the label on the jar because sodium content changes with the type of olives. But olive oil has been more than mere food to the peoples of the Mediterranean; it has been medicinal, magical, as well as a fountain of wealth and power. Between the 7th and 3rd centuries B.C. philosophers, physicians, and historians already referred to its curative properties.

Al: How can oil make people wealthy and powerful?

Emi: Remember we are talking about olive oil—"liquid gold," as it has been named. Olive oil was the hottest commodity in Greece, as it was later on in Rome. In fact, Greek and Roman ships were built for the sole purpose of transporting the oil to trading posts around the Mediterranean. Let me explain first how the oil is produced because the manufacturing process determines quality.

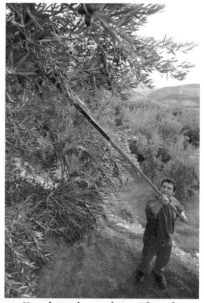

From Olive to Olive Oil

Emi: The harvest of the olive has barely changed over the years. In fact, in many regions, olives are still beaten from the tree with poles and caught in large nets as you can see in this picture. Nowadays, however, many olive farmers use branch shaker machines.

Knocking down olives. Photo by J.A. Sanguinetti. Courtesy of Diputación Provincial de Jaen, Spain.

Al: How interesting!

Emi: Thousands of years ago, the olives were crushed by hand in spherical stone basins. Today, in a similar method, olives (with pits) are pounded and crushed using mechanical techniques. The oil produced in such a way (cold) is the extra virgin olive oil, the natural juice from the olives. It preserves the unique flavor, smell, and healthy properties of the fruit.

Al: The oil we buy at the market is extra virgin?

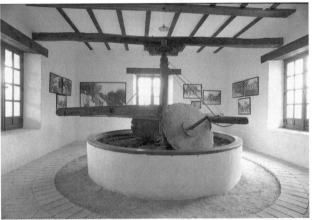

Milling, pressing, and decanting of olives. Photo by Sitoh.
Courtesy of Diputación Provincial de Jaen, Spain.

Emi: Not all of it. The solid residue that remains after the first extraction is sent back to the press to be beaten again and be exposed to different heat levels and chemical procedures. It is neutralized with sodium hydroxide, passed through charcoal filters, and extracted with hexane at low temperatures. The resulting oil lacks color and aroma, and has lost most of its antioxidant properties.

Al: There are a lot of chemicals involved in the processing of this oil!

Emi: True. That's why these second extractions are not recommended for consumption. With time, the use of oils that have been subjected to chemical agents may have a toxic effect on our bodies. (*Pointing at the different bottles of olive* *oil sitting on the table*) These are the kinds of olive oil you can find in the market:

- Extra virgin olive oil, cold pressed
- Virgin olive oil
- Light or mild olive oil

Al: I guess it goes without saying that I should buy extra virgin olive oil, right?

Emi: Correct. It may be a little more expensive, but in the long run you may save a lot of money and a lot of grief. A nine-month study at the University of Granada in Spain compared the effects of extra virgin and refined olive oils on the levels of LDL oxidation in men with *blood vessel disease* (decreased blood flow to the arms and legs due to the thickening and narrowing of the blood vessels). The participants consumed extra virgin olive oil for the first three months. During the next three months they did not consume any olive oil. For the final three months they were given refined oil. The re-sults showed that the amount of LDL oxidation was significantly lower after the patients consumed the extra vir-gin olive oil than after they consumed refined olive oil.[1]

Al: That says a lot in favor of the extra virgin.

Emi: Yes. Do you use olive oil at home?

Al: I think so.

Emi: Do you know what kind?

Al: No. We usually buy the cheapest one. I didn't think the type was important. I see that the oils you have here have differ-ent colors; some are lighter than others. Does the color matter?

Emi: The color of the oil is not indicative of its quality unless it's light and clear as a result of having been refined with chemi-cal agents.

Al: Why is olive oil so good for the heart?

Emi: Two main reasons:

- The main fat in olive oil is monounsaturated.
- Olive oil contains many antioxidants.

You may remember these are two factors that help lower cholesterol.

Al: Yes, I remember but what do you mean by "main fat"?

Fat Composition of Olive Oil

Emi: Last week we saw that the best kind of fat for our heart is monounsaturated because it lowers the "bad" cholesterol, and raises the "good one." (*Showing Al a chart of the fat composition of olive oil*) Look at this chart. Here you can appreciate the proportion of the different fats that make up olive oil:

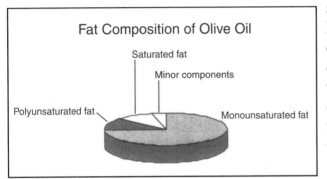

- Oleic acid, monounsaturated: 65 to 80 percent of olive oil
- Linoleic, polyunsaturated: 9 to 10 percent
- Linolenic, polyunsaturated: 0 to 1.5 percent
- Saturated fat: 10 percent
- Minor components (antioxidants): 3 to 4 percent

Al: The monounsaturated portion is really high. Does this mean olive oil does not get stuck in the arteries?

Emi: Right.

Al: It sounds like the perfect oil.

Emi: Well, there is nothing perfect in life, but olive oil comes close. In fact, olive oil has been called "liquid gold" for its exceptional cooking properties, which make it irreplaceable for human consumption. There was a study conducted that included four types of diets for a five-week period: One diet was rich in saturated fats; another one in polyunsaturated fat (sunflower oil); a third in monounsaturated fat (extra virgin olive oil); and the last in omega-3 fatty acids from fish. The study showed that when people followed the diet rich in extra virgin olive oil, the levels of bad cholesterol went down and blood pressure decreased 5 to 6 percent.[2] But the health benefits of olive oil do not end with its high proportion of monounsaturated fat. What makes olive oil really unique are its *minor components*.

Al: What do you mean by "minor components"?

Emi: Compounds found in the oil in small amounts that are very beneficial for our hearts.

The "Minor Components" of Olive Oil

Emi: Countless studies conducted to examine the activities of these minor compounds have indicated that they are strong antioxidants and potent free radical scavengers. They prevent the oxidation of LDL cholesterol, as well as the oxidation of the oil, although with time, of course, oil goes through oxidation and becomes rancid.

Al: When the oil starts tasting and smelling funny it is because it's oxidized?

Emi: Yes. Extra virgin olive oil is a natural product without preservatives and eventually gets oxidized. However, these minor components delay the process. Let's see what these components are.

Vitamin E (α-tocopherol)

Emi: Olive oil contains alpha-tocopherol or vitamin E, the tocopherol with the highest natural antioxidant activity and one of the most effective defenders against oxidation in our cell membranes. Because vitamin E is soluble in fat, the LDL particles carry the vitamin to our cells.

Al: Are you saying that vitamin E is carried inside the same "buses" that deliver cholesterol to our cells?

Emi: Exactly. This means the cholesterol traveling inside the lipoproteins is protected and its level of oxidation is lower. Consistent evidence shows that people with low levels of vitamin E in the blood have more damage in the arteries.[3]

Al: It's amazing the way this vitamin works.

Emi: Yes. On average, the amount of vitamin E in the oil is about 24 to 43 milligrams for each 100 grams of oil.[4] A tablespoon of extra virgin olive oil contains 1.6 milligrams (2.3 IU [International Units]) of vitamin E, providing 8 percent of the recommended daily intake.

Al: I take vitamin E capsules.

Emi: Capsules can never replace the real thing. In the past we have assumed that taking vitamin E supplements would have the same effect as ingesting the vitamin from real foods, but new studies have shown that is not the case. Researchers for the Heart Outcomes Prevention Evaluation Study (HOPE) found that people who received 265 milligrams (400 IU) of vitamin E daily in the form of supplements did not have fewer hospitalizations for heart failure or chest pain when compared to those who received *placebo*, a faked pill. According to this study, people are better off consuming natural vitamin E from foods than from supplements.[5]

Al: Should I stop taking them?

Emi: If the supplement comes in a multivitamin you take every day, you can continue taking it. But if you really want to reap the benefits of vitamin E, you should include olive oil in your diet.

Al: I see.

Polyphenols: tyrosol and hydroxytyrosol

Emi: Polyphenols are potent antioxidants. Extensive research shows that polyphenols are potent inhibitors of free radical "attacks." Tyrosol is quite stable and is able to undo oxidation of LDL cholesterol.[6] Hydroxytyrosol is an efficient trash picker of free radicals and it contributes to the shelf life of the oil, preventing its auto-oxidation.[7] Based on some studies,[8] on average, these compounds in olive oil account for the following approximate levels:

- Extra virgin olive oil: *4.2 milligrams for each 100 grams*
- Refined olive oil: *0.47 milligrams for each 100 grams*

Al: There is a big difference between the amounts found in extra virgin olive oil and refined oils.

Emi: I am glad you noticed that. This is why it is so important to choose extra virgin olive oil. When we buy refined olive oil, most of the antioxidants are gone.

Hydrocarbons: squalene

Emi: The major hydrocarbon in olive oil is *squalene,* a powerful antioxidant. One study[9] shows that the average intake of squalene is 30 milligrams per day in the United States. The intake in the Mediterranean countries can reach 200–400 milligrams per day. The dose of squalene found in olive oil is approximately as follows:

- Extra virgin olive oil: *400–450 milligrams per 100 grams*
- Refined olive oil: *25 percent less than extra virgin oil*[10]

Al: I guess all these differences keep adding up when it comes to protecting our arteries.

Emi: You're right.

Al: At the market, I should just look for extra virgin olive oil?

Emi: Yes. Let me give you a few tips to keep in mind when buying olive oil.

Facts to Keep in Mind When Buying Olive Oil

- Buy "extra virgin olive oil, cold pressed." This is the oil obtained from the first pressing of the fruit and conserves all the vitamins and antioxidant qualities of the olives. Refined olive oil loses most of the original antioxidants during the refining procedures.

- Extra virgin oil can be filtered or unfiltered. Filtration is the process by which microscopic bits from the olive have been removed. Unfiltered oil would be cloudy until it settles to the bottom; it has a deeper flavor because of the fruit.

- Rancidity speeds up when the oil is exposed to light and heat. Buy olive oil in bottles that are dark in color and keep the oil container in the dark, at room temperature.

- The color of olive oil is dependent on the pigments in the fruit, such as chlorophyll and carotenoid. The color of the oil is not indicative of its quality unless it's light as a result of having been refined with chemicals.

- Olive oil does not get better with time. Do not buy very large containers unless you have a large family.

- Check the oil's acidity on the label. Acidity in this case does not refer to the usual meaning "acid" but to the proportion of mono-, poly-, and saturated fatty acids contained in the oil. Guidelines for acidity are as follows:
  - Extra virgin olive oil, with a low degree of acidity, less than 1.0 percent, is a guarantee of a healthy fruit. This classification is based on the European Union standards.
  - Refined olive oils include classifications such as "fine virgin oil" with acidity between 1 and 2 percent.
  - Ordinary virgin olive oil has an acidity range between 2 and 3.3 percent.

Al: How much olive oil do I have to use for it to be effective?

Our Heart Needs a Daily Dose of Olive Oil

Emi: Nutrition authorities recommend 2 to 3 tablespoons of extra virgin olive oil a day as prevention.

Al: Is that the amount Mediterranean people consume?

Emi: No. People in the Mediterranean countries use more, but they also walk more. Remember that olive oil should always replace other sources of fat such as butter and margarine, and not be added to. Butter is rarely consumed in the traditional Mediterranean region and margarine was completely unknown in the area until recently.

Al: I have noticed that some restaurants put a sprig of rosemary or other dried herbs in a bottle of olive oil. Should I do that at home?

Emi: That is based on personal taste. I personally like the plain flavor of the oil. Do you usually fry foods at home?

Al: Sometimes.

Advantages of Frying with Olive Oil

Emi: Although I certainly discourage it, if you do fry foods, be sure to use olive oil. Without overheating, extra virgin olive oil does not change its structure and keeps its nutritional value better than other oils. When heated, olive oil is the most stable fat. Its high smoking point (210 degrees Celsius) is higher than the ideal temperature for frying food (180 degrees Celsius). Fats with lower smoking points, such as corn oil and butter, break down at 180 degrees Celsius temperature and form toxic products. Another advantage to using olive oil for frying is that it forms a crust on the surface of the food that impedes the penetration of oil and improves its flavor. As a result, food fried in olive oil has a lower fat content than food fried in other oils.

Al: That's good to know.

Emi: The International Olive Oil Council[11] recommends the following when frying with olive oil:

- Although the digestibility of heated olive oil does not change when reused for frying several times, it should not be used more than four or five times.
- Olive oil should not be mixed with other fats or vegetable oils.
- The oil used for frying should always be hot; if it is cold, the food will soak up the oil.
- There should always be plenty of oil in the pan when deep frying. If only a small amount is used, not only will it burn more easily but the food being fried will be undercooked on top and overcooked on the bottom.

Al: Is olive oil fattening?

Emi: All oils have 120 calories per tablespoon.

Al: I'm going to stop at the market and surprise my wife with a bottle of the best extra virgin olive oil I can find. I'm sure she is not familiar with all this stuff.

Emi: Excellent. Are you going back to your cooking class tomorrow?

Al: Yes—the kids are looking forward to it. I bought aprons for the children and myself because last time we got our clothes pretty dirty. Oh, I forgot to tell you that since my wife is not working this weekend, I have booked a cabin in the mountains for one night. We leave tomorrow after lunch and come back Sunday night.

Emi: Oh, how wonderful! I'm really envious! Well, have a great weekend, and I'll see you Monday.

REFERENCES

1. Ramirez-Tortosa MC, Urbano G, Lopez Jurado M, Nestares T, Gomez M, Mir A, Ros E, Mataix J, Gil A. Extra-virgin olive oil increases the resistance of LDL to oxidation more than refined olive oil in free-living men with peripheral vascular disease. *Journal of Nutrition.* 1999;129:2177–2183.

2. Montoya MT, Porres A, Serrano S, Fruchart JC, Mata P, Gómez Gerique JA, Rosa Castro G. Fatty acid saturation of the diet and plasma lipid concentrations, lipoprotein particle concentrations, and cholesterol efflux capacity. *American Journal of Clinical Nutrition.* 2002;75:484–491.

3. Psomiadou E, Tsimidou M, Boskou D. Alpha-tocopherol content of Greek virgin olive oils. *Journal of Agricultural and Food Chemistry.* 2000;48:1770–5.

4. See note 3, above.

5. The Heart Outcomes Prevention Evaluation study investigators (HOPE). *New England Journal of Medicine.* 2000;342:145–153.

6. Giovannini C, Straface E, Modesti D, Coni E, Cantafora A, De Vincenzi M, Malorni W, Masella R. Tyrosol, the major olive oil biophenol, protects against oxidized LDL-induced injury in Caco-2 Cells. *Journal of Nutrition.* 1999;129:1269–1277.

7. D'Angelo S, Manna C, Migliardi V, Masón O, Morrica P, Capasso G, Pontoni G, Galletti P, Zappia V. Pharmacokinetics and metabolism of hydroxytyrosol, a natural antioxidant from olive oil. *Drug Metabolism and Disposition.* 2001 Nov;Vol 29, Issue 11, 1492–1498.

8. Owen RW, Mier W, Giacosa A, Hull WE, Spiegelhalder B, Bartsch H. Phenolic compounds and squalene in olive oils: the concentration and antioxidant potential of total phenols, simple phenols, secoiridoids, lignans, and squalene. *Food and Chemical Toxicology.* 2000;38:647–59.

9. Smith TJ. Squalene: potential chemopreventive agent. *Expert Opinion on Investigational Drugs.* 2000;9:1841–8.

10. See note 8, above.

11. www.internationaloliveoil.org.

Chapter Ten

Legumes and Whole Grains: The Cholesterol-Fiber Link

Counseling Session—Day 7
Monday, 4:00 P.M.

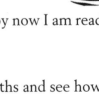

Al: Good afternoon, Emi. How was your weekend?

Emi: Probably not as good as yours. Did you guys have a good time in the mountains?

Al: Fantastic! We walked and walked. I think by now I am ready to take part in the Los Angeles Marathon.

Emi: The enrollment period is still open.

Al (*Rolling his eyes*): I'll wait a couple of months and see how I feel. Who knows? I may join it. The one who seems to be getting in great shape is Napoleon.

Emi: Isn't that wonderful?

Al: Yes, but he is driving me crazy! Do you know that every evening, after I finish dinner, he comes to me holding his leash in his mouth? How on earth does he know when it's time for our daily walk?

Emi: Dogs have a special instinct, and he might be looking forward to seeing his doggy friends. Tell me, how did the cooking class go?

Al: It went really well. I never thought I would enjoy this cooking business so much, especially after all the criticism I received in the past.

Emi: Getting familiar with the "know-how" of cooking makes a difference. What did you make this time?

Al: We prepared Garlic Chicken Breasts and Orange Color Salad.

Emi: Orange color salad? What type of salad is that?

Al: It's made with oranges, carrots, onions, and seasoned with olive oil and lemon. I brought you the recipes.

Emi: Thank you; it sounds really tasty. Okay, now, are you ready to move to today's subject—legumes and grains?

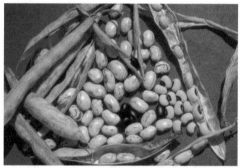

Al: Sure! By legumes you mean dry beans?

Emi: Yes. Legumes include dry beans, lentils, and chickpeas, or garbanzo beans.

Beans of the Old and New World. Photo by Dr. Segundo Rios Ruiz. Courtesy of the Institute of Biodiversity—CIBIO. University of Alicante, Spain.

Al: I see. Are they also good for the heart?

Emi: Very. Based on studies conducted during more than 25 years, nutrition experts at the Michigan State University concluded that eating 2 to 4 cups of cooked dry beans every week can protect us against heart disease.[1] Legumes have been a staple food in the Mediterranean countries for centuries. They are packed with *fiber* as well as minerals and vitamins such as iron, magnesium, manganese, phosphorous, zinc, potassium, *folic acid*, and some of the B-complex vitamins. They are low in fat and sodium, and to top it all, they can help balance your budget because they are very inexpensive. Thus, if legumes are not part of your regular diet, you may be missing an almost perfect food.

Al: If they can help balance my budget they are definitely the perfect food.

Emi: Do you like dry beans?

Al: I have them when I go to Mexican restaurants, so I guess that means "yes." How do they help with heart disease?

Emi: Legumes contain soluble fiber, the type that lowers cholesterol.

Al: I heard about fiber, but to be honest, I don't quite know what it is.

Fiber: A Quick Overview

Emi: Fiber is what gives plants its structure. It's found mainly in fruits, vegetables, legumes, nuts, and seeds, as well as whole grains. It is the portion of plants that our system can not break down because it doesn't have the appropriate mechanisms to do it. Consequently, our cells have very little use for fiber.

Al: Then, why do we care about it?

Emi: Because our bodies, always looking for an intelligent way to use what nature has put at our disposal, have found ways to put fiber to work for us, such as preventing constipation. Fiber can be soluble and insoluble, and most plant foods contain a combination of both. Both types are important for our health, but the fiber that interest us today is the soluble type because is the one that lowers cholesterol.

Al: What does *soluble fiber* mean?

Emi: Soluble fiber means that it dissolves in water and forms a jelly-like paste with other foods in the intestine. This feature is very important, as we'll see, because it reduces the amount of cholesterol circulating in the blood. Soluble fiber not only lowers LDL cholesterol, the "bad" guy, but also raises HDL cholesterol, the "good" guy.

Al: Is insoluble fiber also good for our hearts?

Emi: *Insoluble fiber* is good for our whole body because it acts as a natural laxative. It removes toxic waste by promoting regular bowel movement, but it does not have any effect on cholesterol.

Al: How does soluble fiber lower cholesterol?

Emi: Let me explain.

The Cholesterol-Fiber Link

Emi: *Bile,* produced by the liver, is a substance necessary to break down the fat we ingest in food. To produce bile, the liver gets the cholesterol from the blood, converts it into bile, and sends it to the gallbladder where it's stored until needed. When we eat, the gallbladder sends the bile to the intestines to help break down the fat portion of the food. Once the bile has done its job in the intestines, one of two things can happen:

1. If our meal has enough soluble fiber, the fiber grabs the bile and takes it out of our body through the feces. Once the bile is gone, the liver responds by drawing more cholesterol from the blood to make new bile. The result is less cholesterol circulating in our system.

2. If our meal does not have enough soluble fiber, the bile is not taken out of the body. In this case, the liver doesn't need to draw more cholesterol from the blood to produce more bile because there is plenty available in the system. The result is more cholesterol navigating in our blood vessels.

Emi: There is one more benefit from eating this type of fiber. When our meal includes soluble fiber, it gets fermented by bacteria in the colon. This fermentation produces certain compounds that prevent the formation of cholesterol. This results in lower levels of cholesterol circulating in our blood vessels.

Al: That means less risk for heart attack, right?

Emi: Right. One study examined the relationship between soluble fiber intake and the risk of heart disease on 9,632 men and women over a period of 19 years. It showed that consuming legumes four times or more per week, compared with less than once a week, lowered the risk of heart disease by 22 percent.[2]

Al: Do I need to eat legumes every day?

Emi: You don't have to. Nutrition experts at the University of Michigan recommend two to four cups of legumes a week to reduce the risk of heart disease.[3] Try to include a variety of legumes. Another benefit of including legumes as part of your diet is the effect they have on *homocysteine.*

Al: What is that?

What Is Homocysteine?

Emi: Homocysteine is a substance our body needs to produce certain compounds vital for our organs to function properly. To produce homocysteine, our bodies need adequate amounts of vitamin B6, B12, and folic acid. When any of these vitamins is lacking, homocysteine is not converted into the necessary compounds and spills into the circulation. Many studies have shown that when homocysteine accumulates in our system, it becomes toxic even in small amounts, increasing the risk of heart disease. High levels of homocysteine concentrations in our blood may cause a heart attack or a stroke, even among people who have normal cholesterol levels.

Al: How can homocysteine cause heart attacks?

Emi: Abnormal levels of homocysteine appear to:

- Damage the inner lining of the arteries
- Promote blood clots
- Oxidize LDL cholesterol

Al: First time I've heard this term.

Emi: It's not common, but a lot of research is being done in this area.

Al: What do I do to prevent homocysteine from accumulating in my blood?

Emi: Eat foods that contain folate as well as vitamins B6 and B12. Legumes are an excellent source of folate and contain moderate amounts of B6. Recent data show that the practice of fortifying foods with folate has reduced the average level of homocysteine in the U.S. population. Let's talk now about whole grains.

Whole Grains

Al: What do you mean by "whole" grains?

Emi: Whole grains are the entire seed of a plant. The seed is made of three parts: the *bran*, the *germ*, and the *endosperm*.

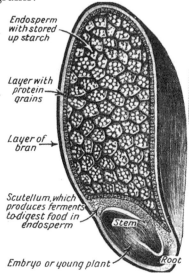

Endosperm with stored up starch

Layer with protein grains

Layer of bran

Scutellum, which produces ferments to digest food in endosperm

Stem

Embryo or young plant

Root

- *Bran.* The outer layer, a kind of skin that protects the kernel, contains important antioxidants, B vitamins, and fiber.

- *Germ.* The embryo, which would sprout into a new plant, contains many B vitamins, some protein, minerals, and healthy fats.

- *Endosperm.* The largest portion of the kernel, it contains carbohydrates, proteins, and small amounts of vitamins and minerals.

As you can see, whole grains contribute a good amount of soluble and insoluble fiber, antioxidants, as well as B vitamins, vitamin E, magnesium, and iron.

Al: I thought all grains were whole.

Emi: No. The white bread you see at the market is made from wheat flour from which the bran and germ have been removed.

Al: When the bran and the germ are removed it makes a difference in the amount of vitamins and fiber we get, right?

White or Brown Bread—Does It Make a Difference?

Emi: A big difference. Without the bran and the germ, about 25 percent of the grain's protein is lost, along with at least 17 key nutrients. In addition, white flour is generally bleached using potassium bromate or chlorine dioxide gas to remove any yellow color.

Al: Ugh! I need to buy brown bread, right?

Emi: You have to be careful because not every brown bread is made with 100 percent whole grains.

Brown Doesn't Mean It Is Whole Grain

Emi: Most "whole wheat" or "brown" bread produced in the United States is primarily made of bleached white flour with the addition of enough brown flour to make it look brown.

Al: How can I tell if the product is whole grain?

Emi: The food label is the best tool to find out about a product. Look for words such as "100% whole grain" or "100% whole wheat." Check the list of ingredients. If the first ingredient listed is "whole wheat flour" or "whole oats," most likely the product is whole grain. Currently, manufacturers can also indicate on food labels the amount of grams contained in the product such as "10 grams of whole grains" or "½ ounce of whole grains." Statements such as "whole grain" or "made with whole grain" may contain very small amounts of whole grains.

The Whole Grains Council has created a packaging symbol called the "whole grain stamp." The 100 percent stamp assures you that a food contains a full serving of whole grain in each serving and that all the grain is whole grain.[4]

Al: Why are whole grains important for our hearts?

Why Are Whole Grains Important for Our Hearts?

Emi: For the same reasons legumes are. Some grains are high in soluble fiber, which lowers cholesterol.

Al: What grains have soluble fiber?

Emi: Grains that have a high amount of soluble fiber are oats, barley, quinoa, and psyllium husks.

Al: You mean, "oats" as in oatmeal?

Emi: Yes.

Al: I am already eating it! I told my wife what you said about oatmeal being good for high blood pressure and the brand you recommended, and since then she has being making oatmeal in the mornings. She cooks it with a stick of cinnamon and 1 percent lowfat milk. It tastes really good!

Emi: I had no idea you were having such a healthy breakfast. Congratulations!

Al: Thank you. How much soluble fiber will lower cholesterol?

Emi: Scientific studies published in the *Journal of the American Medical Association* and the *American Journal of Public Health* have shown that it takes 3 grams of oat-soluble fiber per day to reduce cholesterol levels. How much are you eating now?

Al: My wife uses ½-cup of oatmeal for each of us.

Emi: That provides you with 3 grams of soluble fiber daily. Health authorities recommend ingesting 25 to 35 grams of fiber a day, including both soluble and insoluble. About 6 to 10 grams should be soluble. This level is easy to achieve with the recommended six or more servings of whole grains.

Al: How much is a serving of grains?

Emi: A serving is one slice of bread, ½ cup of oats, or ⅓ cup of brown rice.

Al: I never had the faintest idea about this whole grain business. In fact, I thought the whiter, the better. There is a bakery near my house; I'll have to check and see what kinds of bread they have.

Emi: If all you ate were white bread, white rice, white pasta, and so on, your organs would be deprived of many vitamins they need.

Al: I have one last question. Last Saturday, our cooking teacher asked us to bring a recipe of our choice to class. Do you think it would be a good idea to bring one that includes legumes?

Emi: Absolutely! Do you have anything in mind or would you like a suggestion?

Al: I would like a suggestion, if you don't mind.

Emi: It will be a pleasure to help you. How about a bean salad and hummus? They are very easy to make and would be appropriate given the theme of the class.

Al: Sounds good.

Emi: I'm also going to give you a garbanzo bean salad recipe; it's one of my favorites. As you know, tomorrow is our last counseling session in this series of meetings. We'll cover garlic and onions, and then we'll review any areas where you may need some clarification.

Al: You know, I'm going to miss our discussions. I don't know if you have the time Wednesday, but my wife and I would like to take you out to dinner after we are done here. She has changed her daily hours, and she would join us with the children at the restaurant. They all want to meet you.

Emi: I'd be delighted to have dinner with your family. Tell them I'll be looking forward to meeting them.

Al: I'll let them know. They are thinking about having dinner at an Italian restaurant. Would that be alright with you?

Emi: It would be perfect.

Al: I'll make the reservations. See you Wednesday.

REFERENCES

1. www.michiganstateuniversity.org.
2. Bazzano L, He J, Ogden L, Loria C, Suma Vupputuri S, Myers L, Whelton P, Legume consumption and risk of coronary heart disease in US men and women. *Archives of Internal Medicine.* 2001;161:2573–2578 (a).
3. See note 1, above.
4. www.wholegrainscouncil.org/research.htm.

Orange Color Salad

Makes 2 servings

Ingredients

4 large carrots
1 small onion
1 large orange
1 lemon
3 tablespoons extra virgin olive oil

Preparation

Wash the carrots and onions, and grate them. Place them in a bowl. Peel the orange, remove the seeds, and cut in small pieces. In a small bowl, beat the lemon juice and olive oil until it becomes a homogeneous mixture. Pour over the ingredients and serve cold.

Chicken Breasts

Makes 4 servings

Ingredients

4 chicken breast halves
1 clove of garlic
salt
black pepper
extra virgin olive oil

Preparation

The chicken breasts should be very thin, cut butterfly style or pounded. Cut the clove of garlic in half and rub both sides of the chicken with the garlic. Season the breasts with a pinch of salt, black pepper, and olive oil. Cook in a nonstick fry pan for two or three minutes on each side.

Hummus

Makes 4 to 6 servings, approximately

Ingredients

2 garlic cloves
2 lemons
1 6-ounce can chickpeas
4 tablespoons tahini
pinch of salt
2 tablespoons olive oil
pinch of paprika

Preparation

Peel and chop the garlic, and squeeze the juice from the lemons. Put everything (except the paprika) into a blender, and blend until smooth. Add a little water, if necessary. Pour into a dish and sprinkle with the paprika. Serve as a dip with pita pockets.

Bean Salad

Makes 6 servings

Ingredients

> 2 16-ounce cans mixed beans (navy, cannellini,
>   black-eyed peas, red kidney beans, etc.)
> ½ pound green beans, trimmed
> 6–8 green onions, chopped

Dressing

> juice of 1 lemon
> 2–3 tablespoons wine vinegar
> 4 large cloves garlic, minced
> ½ cup extra virgin olive oil
> black pepper

Preparation

Drain canned beans and rinse thoroughly. Steam green beans until just tender. Toss all beans together with the green onions.

In a small bowl, mix the lemon juice, vinegar, garlic, olive oil, and black pepper, and add to the beans. Toss again. Serve at room temperature.

Chickpea and Olive Salad

Makes 4 servings

Ingredients

1 15-ounce can chickpeas, drained
1 small cucumber
2 medium tomatoes
1 small red onion
3 tablespoons chopped fresh parsley
½ cup pitted black olives
1 tablespoon lemon juice
3 tablespoons extra virgin olive oil
1 teaspoon honey

Preparation

Drain chickpeas. Cut cucumber and tomatoes in small cubes, and chop onion fine. Combine chickpeas, cucumber, tomatoes, onion, parsley, and olives in a bowl. Place lemon, olive oil, and honey in a small jar and shake well. Pour over the salad.

Chapter Eleven

Garlic Can Protect Us From More Than Vampires

Emi: How did it go today?

Al: Pretty good.

Emi: Are you and your family going to the mountains this weekend?

Al: No. Next Saturday is my brother-in-law's birthday, so I'm having a party for him.

Emi: Planning on buying a big cake?

Al: I'm going to buy a fruit tart, and the children and I will make oatmeal cookies.

Emi: I'm very impressed! You could put some chocolate chips in your cookies.

Al That's not a bad idea. (*In a sheepish voice*) I'm also buying ice cream for dessert.

Emi: Nothing wrong with that as long as you have it only on special occasions. As you know, today is our last day, and we are going to talk about two very important herbs in the Mediterranean diet: garlic and onions.

Al (*Looking with amazement at some garlic bulbs*): Garlic is also beneficial for the heart?

Emi: Yes. This herb is very important in the fight against heart disease.

Al: That's right! I remember you mentioned garlic during our first discussion as one of the pillars of the Mediterranean diet.

Emi: Exactly.

Garlic, a Wonder of Nature

Emi: Garlic is truly a wonder of nature. More than 200 chemical compounds that might protect our bodies have been found in garlic. Lately, scientists and nutrition experts are paying close attention to this herb because it has shown it can reduce cholesterol and triglycerides, lower blood pressure, and prevent the formation of blood clots. It can also protect our arteries through its antioxidant properties.

Al: It's hard to believe a couple of garlic cloves can have such an effect on the body.

Emi: Well, it takes more than a couple of cloves to reap the benefits of garlic, but you may find it interesting to know that garlic has been used for thousand of years as both food and medicine. People around the world, especially those who enjoy few chronic diseases, use garlic extensively in their daily diets.

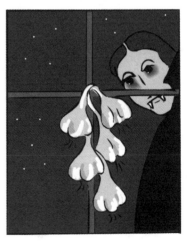

Al: Is it true that in the past people would rub garlic on doors and windows to ward off vampires?

Emi: Yes.

Al: Why did people do such a strange thing?

Emi: Hard to tell, although in this case there are several theories. One of them holds that a vampire's bite is seen as a mosquito sting, and garlic is known in folklore as a natural mosquito repellent. Mosquitoes suck blood and in doing so, they spread disease. So do vampires. Of course, the 64,000-dollar question is, can garlic keep vampires at bay? Let's hope we never have to find out.

Al: I agree.

Emi: Although modern research has not confirmed yet that rubbing garlic on doorknobs and window frames can protect us against vampires or evil spirits, it has confirmed what our ancestors believed about the health benefits of this herb: its consumption can protect us from many ailments.

Al: Has garlic really been used as a medicine in the past?

Emi: Yes. In 1858, Louis Pasteur demonstrated that garlic has antibiotic properties and can kill infectious bacteria. Garlic was used throughout World War I to treat battle wounds and to cure dysentery. During World War II, when penicillin was scarce or not available, the British and Russian armies used garlic to cure wound infections and prevent *gangrene*; it came to be known as "Russian penicillin."

Al: Why isn't garlic used as medicine anymore?

Emi: Unfortunately, for several decades, the widespread use of antibiotics has ignored the medical properties of garlic. Lately, however, interest in garlic has escalated and nowadays research is focusing on the role garlic plays in the prevention and control of heart disease.

Al: Does garlic really help in the treatment of heart disease?

Emi: Many studies show it does.

Al: How?

Emi: In several ways.

Garlic and High Blood Pressure

Emi: High blood pressure is one of the health conditions where garlic treatment brings the fastest results.

Al: But how does garlic do that?

Emi: Studies suggest that garlic dilates blood vessel walls, increasing the diameter of the arteries. Garlic also helps to prevent high blood pressure by preventing blood cells from sticking together. In a clinical trial, the subjects ingested standardized garlic powder capsules for four years.[1] The results showed a 9 to 18 percent reduction in plaque volume and a 7 percent decrease in blood pressure. This resulted in an increase in the diameter of the arteries by 4 percent, which is associated with an 18 percent improvement of blood flow. These effects of garlic resulted in a risk reduction for heart attacks and strokes by more than 50 percent.[1]

Al: Did you also say that garlic is good to lower cholesterol?

Garlic Can Lower Your Blood Cholesterol

Emi: Yes. Studies indicate that the populations that eat garlic consistently have the lowest level of blood cholesterol. Pennsylvania State University showed that men with high total blood cholesterol were able to lower its concentration by 7 percent and LDL by 10 percent when taking garlic supplements. The study indicated that the sulfur compounds in garlic were responsible for the results, especially S-allylcysteine, which inhibits the formation of cholesterol by the liver.[2] Flinders University of South Australia conducted a review of 16 studies carried out with 952 subjects. The review showed that the participants who went through garlic therapy achieved a 12 percent reduction in their cholesterol levels. The reduction was evident after one month of therapy and continued for at least six months. The researchers used a dose of dried garlic powder oscillating between 600 and 900 milligrams daily. The same studies showed that dried garlic powder preparations lowered trig-lycerides.[3]

Al: I guess I will have to start eating garlic! By the way, what are *platelets?*

Garlic and Platelets

Emi: Platelets are tiny cells in the blood that, when arteries get damaged, rush to the lesion site to repair them.

Al: How do they repair them?

Emi: They become sticky and form a clot. Unfortunately, although platelets' intentions are good, these clots are the first step toward the formation of a *thrombus*, an accumulation of plate-lets and protein. A thrombus may in time obstruct the flow of blood in the blood vessels.

Al: Can a thrombus cause a heart attack?

Emi: Yes. A thrombus usually stays attached to the blood vessel, but it can break loose and travel through the bloodstream. It can move to the brain, causing a stroke; to the heart, causing a heart attack; or to other parts of the body. No matter where the thrombus goes, it spells trouble.

Al: It sounds dangerous.

Emi: Very. And here is where garlic comes to the rescue. Studies have shown that small doses of garlic can prevent platelets from becoming sticky and piling up together.

Al: This garlic seems pretty powerful. How does it do that?

Emi: By blocking the formation of a compound that causes the formation of a thrombus. In a study carried out by Liverpool John Moores University, the subjects experienced a reduc-tion of platelet stickiness after ingesting 5 milliliters of garlic extract per day for 13 weeks.[4]

Al: Amazing!

Garlic and Plaque in the Arteries

Emi: The formation of plaque is another area where garlic can help. As we have already seen, plaque starts to form when arteries are damaged. Plaque keeps growing and with time may block the flow of blood in the arteries.

Al: Yes, I know. I remember you said plaque is made up of mounds of fat and debris deposited in the wall of the arteries that reduce the space available for blood to circulate.

Emi: Exactly. Studies conducted on rabbits have shown that when garlic is eaten regularly, not only does it prevent the formation of plaque but it also dissolves the plaque already formed. One study showed that continuous intake of high doses of garlic powder capsules for four years reduced the plaque volume by 5 to 18 percent. It is also a fact that most people between 50 and 80 years of age have an increase in the amount of plaque. During the four years this study lasted, the volume of plaque remained constant in people within this age frame demonstrating that garlic has a preventive as well as a curative role in heart disease.[5]

Al: It's hard to believe that something as small as garlic cloves can cover so much.

Emi: And we are not done yet. Garlic can also decrease the oxidation of red blood cells in patients with damage in the arteries.

Garlic as an Antioxidant

Emi: Garlic has been shown to protect blood vessels from the destructive effects of free radicals. Ankara University of Turkey conducted a study to investigate the effects of garlic extract on the oxidation of red blood cells. For six months, 11 patients with atherosclerosis ingested a daily dose of 1 milliliter of garlic extract per kilogram of body weight. The study showed a reduction on the level of oxidation of red blood cells in the patients.[6]

Al: There must be a secret why garlic works this way.

Emi: The "secret," as you call it, is a chemical factory that nature has packaged in garlic.

Al: What do you mean by a "chemical factory"?

Emi: I mean that dozens of compounds such as sulfur and selenium have been identified in garlic. These compounds are responsible for many of its medicinal properties and may have been developed by the plant to protect itself from unfriendly animals or even soil-born organisms. To give you an idea, these are just a few of the components in garlic:

- Thirty-three compounds containing sulfur. Among them we find alliin, allicin, cycroalliin, diallyl disulphide, and diallyl trisulphide.
- Minerals such as calcium, copper, iron, potassium, magnesium, selenium, and zinc.
- Vitamin A, B1, and C.

To get the medicinal properties of fresh garlic, however, you must follow a "protocol" before consuming it.

Al: Did you say a protocol?

Emi: Yes. What I mean is that you have to follow several steps before using fresh garlic to obtain its medicinal effects. Let me show you.

Cooking Garlic Involves a "Protocol"

Emi (*Grabbing a garlic bulb*): First peel the cloves, cut them in small pieces, and crush them in a mortar like this (*Showing Al the mortar and pestle sitting on the table*). After you have crushed the garlic, let it sit uncovered in the mortar for 10 or 15 minutes before you put it in the food.

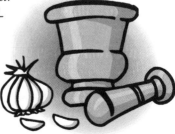

Al: Why?

Emi: The cloves of raw garlic contain alliin. When alliin comes into contact with alliinase, an enzyme found also in the cloves, alliin is converted into allicin. Because alliin and the enzyme alliinase are in different compartments in the garlic cloves, the only way they can come into contact with each other is when the cloves are crushed.

Al: Why is it so important for alliin to be converted into allicin?

Emi: Because once allicin is formed, it triggers other compounds necessary to unleash the medicinal properties of garlic. This process takes about 10 to 15 minutes.

Al: How interesting!

Emi: Two more things to remember when cooking with garlic: First, do not put whole garlic cloves in the food without first crushing them because the heat will destroy the enzyme and as a result, alliin will not be converted into allicin.

Al: That means the garlic will not have any medicinal properties, right?

Emi: Right. The second thing to remember when using garlic in cooked food is to add the garlic last since its active compounds evaporate under intense heat.

Al: I'll follow your indications but my problem with garlic is the odor. Of course I want to take care of my health but I also want to keep my friends, which I am not too sure I can if I start eating a lot of garlic. What do you suggest?

Emi: You can do several things:

Garlic, the Stinking "Rose"

- Eat some fresh parsley or peppermint oil after eating a meal containing garlic; it seems to block the pungent smell caused by allicin.
- Hang around with friends who like garlic.
- Join the local garlic lovers' club.

- Cook your "garlic specials" for your friends and family. I am pretty sure they will love it, and you may be able to start your own garlic lover's club.
- As a last resort, you can move to Italy or Spain. There, you can indulge yourself in garlic and still have lots of friends.

Al: You know, that's not a bad idea! How about if I buy garlic pills, would that help with the odor?

Emi: Yes.

Garlic Supplements

Emi: Garlic supplements may take care of the strong garlic odor, but remember that pills can never replace the fresh product since humans have not been able to carbon-copy nature yet.

Al: If I buy garlic pills, which kind should I get?

Emi: Garlic products are made from fresh or dried garlic cloves but not all garlic pills contain the same amount of active ingredients; in fact, there is a wide variation in the amount of allicin and other important compounds among the different brands. The amount of active compounds present depends on where the garlic is grown, how the product is prepared, and whether it is grown organically or with chemicals. These differences probably explain why the results from scientific studies differ on how well the product lowers cholesterol or improves blood pressure. Buy one that is standardized to ensure you are getting a specific concentration of allicin and other active substances.

Al: What does "standardized" mean?

Emi: It means that a substance contains a guaranteed amount of a certain botanical component. Look for a product that has a high content of allicin. A major concern with garlic supplements is that the amount of compounds containing sulfur or the total allicin potential may not be enough.

Al: What dosage should I be looking for?

Emi: Based on the results obtained from different clinical trials, the dosage should provide a daily dose of at least 10 milligrams of alliin. This dose has the potential to become 4,000 mcg of allicin, roughly the equivalent to one clove of fresh garlic.

Al: Do people in the Mediterranean countries eat garlic every day?

Emi: Pretty much. Fresh garlic is a basic ingredient in almost every meal.

Al: Do they take garlic pills?

Emi: I never met anybody who did. It is hard to imagine Italians or Spaniards taking garlic pills when most of the dishes are prepared with fresh garlic. However, there may be people who use them for different reasons.

Al: How much garlic do I need to take to lower my cholesterol?

Emi: I will list guidelines for you to follow.

Dosage—How Much?

- *Whole garlic clove:* two to three fresh garlic cloves daily, the equivalent of 2 to 4 grams. Each clove is approximately 1 gram.
- *Capsules or tablets:* Take 600 to 900 milligrams of garlic once a day, standardized to 1.3 percent alliin or 0.6 percent allicin. For high cholesterol, high blood pressure, and heart disease prevention, take 600 to 900 milligrams of garlic once or twice a day.

Al: Does raw garlic have any side effects?

Emi: Not really, but let me outline the Commission E advice on garlic for you.

Contraindications and Adverse Effects of Garlic

Emi: The German Government's Commission E, which represents the most accurate information available in the world today on the efficacy of herbs, has reported no known adverse effects with the use of raw garlic. The Commission has approved the use of garlic as a nonprescription medicine to lower cholesterol and triglycerides and as a preventive measure against changes that occur in the blood vessels as we age. Some studies conducted on the use of garlic indicate the following:

- The ingestion of two to four cloves of raw garlic per day is considered safe for adults.
- The most common side effect of ingested garlic is breath and body odor.
- High intakes of raw garlic, especially on an empty stomach, can cause heartburn, flatulence, and in rare instances, mild gastrointestinal symptoms.
- Garlic consumption may increase the anticoagulant effect of Warfarin, a medication prescribed to thin the blood.
- High doses of garlic may increase the effects of blood-thinning medications such as aspirin, vitamin E, and fish oil.
- It is recommended to stop taking high amounts of fresh garlic—more than two cloves a day—or not to exceed the dose indicated on the container (if you are taking garlic pills) seven to ten days before surgery since it can prolong bleeding time.
- Garlic use is not recommended during breastfeeding.

Al: Why not? Is it harmful to the baby?

Emi: No, but it can change the taste of the mother's milk and the baby may not like it. Let me say something briefly about onions, another pillar of the Mediterranean diet.

Al: Are they also good for the heart?

Emi: Yes, onions are highly recommended to prevent heart disease.

Al: Do they work like garlic?

Emi: Very similar. Onions are also members of the allium family. They contain about 25 active compounds that appear to help combat heart disease, strokes, and lower blood pressure and cholesterol.

Al: They have the same kind of compounds as garlic?

Emi: Yes. Yellow and red varieties are abundant in two antioxidants: sulfur and quercetin. Quercetin is also found in red wine but in much lower quantities.

Al: I like raw onions, but again, there goes my social life!

Emi: Most health professionals recommend eating raw onions for maximum benefit but cooking doesn't reduce their potency that much. In fact, unlike sulfur compounds, quercetin can withstand the heat of cooking.

Al: You know, I have seen a place not too far from my house where I think I can get a mortar. I'm going to buy one because I want to start using garlic the right way.

Emi: Excellent move. Well, Al, we have come to the end of our sessions. Is there anything I can clarify for you or that you would like me to elaborate a little further?

Al: One thing I want to say before I go is that I'm very happy my doctor sent me here. Now I know that some of my behaviors have contributed to my high cholesterol and my high blood pressure, and I'm willing to work on correcting them.

Emi: It has been a pleasure working with you, Al. During these weeks you have made an incredible progress. What do you think has motivated you to make the changes you have made?

Al: As we went through our sessions, I realized my lifestyle was reckless. When I became aware that my daily habits may have caused many of the health problems I'm experiencing now, I felt a responsibility to change those habits and take care of myself. I have seen many people around me take tons of pills or go through surgery, and I don't want that life for myself.

Emi: I'm impressed at your motivation; I have learned a lot about determination in watching you. Bear in mind also that there may be times when you might find it tough to change some of your day-to-day habits. The important thing to remember is that if one day you deviate from your good habits, it's no big deal as long as you get back on track the next day. You now have a powerful tool at your disposal: the knowledge of which foods to emphasize and which to limit or avoid. You also have another powerful tool that is as important as having healthy eating habits: the support network you have built around you with your family and friends, including Napoleon. Before we leave, I want to give you a small present I know you will put to some use: a Mediterranean cookbook.

Al: Thank you very much. (*Glancing at some of the pictures*) It's very colorful!

Emi: The Mediterranean cuisine is one of the most colorful cuisines in the world.

Al: What has impressed me from this diet is how each food complements the other.

Emi: You're right. The Mediterranean diet is a synergy of health and aesthetics, and although each component of this diet contributes with an array of benefits on its own, it's the combination of all of them that makes this diet so powerful.

Al: Yes. I must say that through our discussions I have learned to appreciate the Mediterranean diet and its benefits.

Emi: Your body will appreciate it too.

Al: I know. If it's okay with you, we can leave now. I made a reservation at 6:30 P.M. and my wife and the children are probably waiting for us.

Emi: Perfect; let's go. (*Emi closes the door behind them as they leave for the restaurant.*)

REFERENCES

1. Siegel G, Walter A, Engel S, Walper A, Michel F. Pleiotropic effects of garlic. *Wiener Medizinische Wochenschrift.* 1999;149(8–10):217–24.

2. Yeh YY, Liu L. Cholesterol-lowering effect of garlic extracts and organosulfur compounds: human and animal studies. *Journal of Nutrition.* 2001 Mar;131(3s):989S–93S. Department of Nutrition, The Pennsylvania State University, University Park, PA 16802, USA.

3. Silagy CA, Neil HA. Garlic as a lipid lowering agent, a meta-analysis. *Junior Royal College of Physicians of London.* 1994 Jan–Feb;28(1):39–45.

4. Rahman K, Billington D. Dietary supplementation with aged garlic extract inhibits ADP-induced platelet aggregation in humans. *Journal of Nutrition.* 2000 Nov;130(11):2662–5.

5. Koscielny J, Klussendorf D, Latza R, Schmitt R, Radtke H, Siegel G, Kiesewetter H. The antiatherosclerotic effect of Allium sativum. *Atherosclerosis.* 1999 May;144(1):237–49. Comment in: *Atherosclerosis.* 2000 Jun;150(2):437–8.

6. Durak I, Aytac B, Atmaca Y, Devrim E, Avci A, Erol C, Oral D. Effects of garlic extract consumption on plasma and erythrocyte antioxidant parameters in atherosclerotic patients. *Life Sciences.* 2004 Sep 3;75(16):1959–66.

Glossary

A

Aneurysm: the ballooning of an artery.

Antioxidant: a substance in food that protects other substances from oxidation by oxidizing themselves, thus decreasing the adverse effects of free radicals on normal physiological functions in the human body.

Arrhythmia: an irregularity in the normal rhythm or force of the heartbeat.

Arteries: blood vessels that carry blood away from the heart.

Atherosclerosis: the buildup of fatty material in the artery of the walls. The inner lining of the arteries becomes thick and irregular due to the buildup of plaque, which narrows the lumen of the artery and restricts blood flow to the tissue it supplies.

Atom: the smallest portion into which an element can be divided and still retain its properties.

B

Bile acids (bile): a yellowish green fluid produced in the liver, stored in the gallbladder, and sent to the small intestine to process fats.

Blood pressure: the force created by the heart as it pushes blood into the arteries and the circulatory system.

Blood vessels disease: decreased blood flow to the arms and legs due to the thickening and narrowing of blood vessels.

Bran: the husks of cereal grain that are partly or completely removed during the milling process.

C

Calcium: a soft silver-white element that is an alkaline earth metal constituting about three percent of the earth's crust.

Cardiovascular disease (CVD): a general term for all diseases of the heart and blood vessels. Atherosclerosis is the main cause of CVD. When the arteries that carry blood to the heart muscle become blocked, the heart suffers damage known as coronary heart disease (CHD).

Cholesterol: a chemical compound manufactured in the body, used to build cell membranes and brain and nerve tissues. Cholesterol is also used by the body to make steroid hormones and bile acids.

Coronary heart disease or coronary artery disease: disease involving the network of blood vessels surrounding and serving the heart; manifested in clinical end points of myocardial infarction and sudden death.

Chronic: having long duration.

D

Diabetes: a group of metabolic disorders that result from inadequate or ineffective insulin causing abnormal glucose regulation and utilization.

Diastolic blood pressure: blood pressure during the relaxation phase of the cardiac cycle; 80 mm Hg (millimeters of mercury) is optimal.

E

Electron: a stable negatively charged particle that is a constituent of matter and orbits the nucleus of an atom.

Endosperm: the tissue that surrounds the embryo inside a plant seed and provides nourishment for it.

Endothelium: a layer of cell that lines the inside of blood vessels and other body cavities.

Enzyme: a protein produced by the cells that helps in biochemical reactions.

F

Fats: lipids in foods or the body; composed mostly of triglycerides.

Fiber: the coarse fibrous substances in grains, fruits, and vegetables that aid digestion and clean out the intestines.

Folic acid: a vitamin of the B complex, found in green vegetables, fruit, and liver.

Free radicals: a highly reactive atom or group of atoms with an impaired electron.

G

Gangrene: local death and decay of soft tissues of the body as a result of lack of blood supply to the area.

Germ: the embryo in a seed that would sprout into a new plant.

H

Heart attack: a sudden, serious, painful, and sometimes fatal interruption of the heart's normal functioning especially due to a blockage in the coronary artery.

Hemorrhagic stroke: Excessive bleeding. The loss of blood from a ruptured blood vessel, either internally or externally.

High blood pressure: Abnormally high blood pressure in the arteries.

High density lipoprotein: lipoproteins that have more protein than fat. Also known as HDL cholesterol.

Homocysteine: an amino acid, derived from proteins in the diet that can build up in the blood and contribute to the development of heart disease.

Hormone: A chemical substance produced in the endocrine glands or certain other cells that regulates or stimulates bodily functions.

Hydrogenated oil: a fat that has been chemically altered by the addition of hydrogen atoms.

Hydrogenation: the process of inserting hydrogen molecules in liquid vegetable oils.

Hypertension: blood pressure that is dangerously high.

I

Insoluble fiber: fiber incapable of dissolving in water.

L

Lipoproteins: a chemical compound made of fat and protein. A diverse class of particles containing varying amounts of triglyceride, cholesterol, phospholipids, and protein that solubilize lipids for blood transport.

Low-density lipoproteins: lipoproteins that have more fat than protein. Also known as LDL cholesterol. High levels are associated with increased risk of coronary heart disease.

Lycopene: a powerful antioxidant of the carotenoid group found in tomatoes and used in many antioxidant dietary supplements.

M

Magnesium: a cation within the body's cells, active in many enzyme systems.

Mediterranean diet: Refers to nutritional patterns found in countries along the Mediterranean basin where lifestyle has historically been associated with good health.

Metabolism: the total sum of all chemical reactions that go on in living cells.

Microbe: A microscopic organism, especially one that transmits a disease.

Minor components of olive oil: compounds found in small amounts in olive oil that are strong antioxidants and potent free radical scavengers.

Molecule: the smallest physical unit of a substance that can exist independently, consisting of one or more atoms held together by chemical forces.

Monounsaturated fat: a fat composed of triglycerides in which most of the molecules are monounsaturated. Monounsaturated fats tend to lower levels of LDL cholesterol in the blood.

N

Nightshade: A wild plant related to potatoes, tomatoes, and eggplant. Some are poisonous, like deadly nightshade or belladonna.

O

Omega-3 oils: a type of polyunsaturated fat that our body needs to perform certain bodily functions but cannot manufacture or can only manufacture in insufficient amounts.

Organic: produced without the use of synthetic chemicals in favor of naturally occurring pesticides, fertilizers, and other growing aids.

Oxidants: compounds (such as oxygen itself) that oxidize other compounds.

Oxidation: the process of a substance combining with oxygen.

Oxidized LDL cholesterol: A substance formed when the cholesterol in LDL particles is oxidized by free radicals. It is key in the development of atherosclerosis.

Oxidative damage: continuous damage caused by free radicals.

Oxidative stress: a condition in which the production of oxidants and free radicals exceeds the body's ability to defend itself and prevent damage.

P

Pedometer: step counter.

Phytochemical: nonnutrient plant chemical that contain protective, disease-preventing compounds.

Placebo: a drug containing no active ingredients given to a patient participating in a clinical trial in order to assess the performance of a new drug.

Plaque: mounds of lipid material (mostly cholesterol) with some macrophages (a type of white blood cell) covered with fibrous connective tissue and embedded in artery walls. With time, the plaque may harden as the fibrous coat thickens and calcium is deposited in the plaque.

Platelets: a tiny colorless disk-shaped particle found in large quantities in the blood that plays an important part in the clotting process. Platelets' clumping together is one of several steps in blood clotting that can lead to a heart attack.

Polyunsaturated fat: a fat made of polyunsaturated molecules. Poly-unsaturated fats tend to lower levels of both HDL cholesterol and LDL cholesterol in the blood.

Potassium: the principal cation within the body's cells; critical to the maintenance of fluid balance, nerve transmissions, and muscle contraction.

S

Saturated fat: a fat composed of triglycerides in which most of the fatty acids are saturated. Saturated fats tend to raise levels of LDL cholesterol in the blood.

Siesta: short nap, usually in the afternoon.

Sodium: the principal cation in the extra-cellular fluids of the body; critical to the maintenance of fluid balance, nerve transmissions, and muscle contractions.

Soluble fiber: able to dissolve in another substance. It forms a jelly-like paste in the intestine with other foods.

Stroke: a sudden blockage or rupture of a blood vessel in the brain resulting in, for example, loss of consciousness, partial loss of movement, or loss of speech.

Systolic blood pressure: blood pressure during the contraction phase of the cardiac cycle; 120 millimeters of mercury is optimal.

T

Thrombosis: the formation of a thrombus.

Thromboxane: a potent inducer of platelet aggregation.

Thrombus: a clot; an aggregation of platelets and protein, which, if small, can contribute to the growth of plaque and, if large, can obstruct a blood vessel, resulting in angina, myocardial infarction, or sudden death.

Trans fats: a fat composed of triglycerides in which most of the molecules have an unusual configuration around the double bonds.

Triglycerides: the chief form of fat in the diet and the major storage form of fat in the body; composed of a molecule of glycerol with three fatty acids attached. It can refer both to the main form of fat in food or in the body.

V

Vitamins: organic substances essential in small quantities to the nutrition and normal bodily functions of most animals.

W

Whole grain: grains that have the entire seed of a plant.

Index

acids, bile, 83, 137, 138
    definition of, 137
activity, physical:
    direct effects on heart disease,
        16–17
    importance of, 13–22
allium compounds, 55–56
American Diabetes Association, 72
American Heart Association, 76
aneurysm, definition of, 25, 137
antioxidant supplements, 56,
antioxidants, 48–49, 53, 54–56, 60,
    62, 89, 99, 101, 102, 104, 105,
    114, 124–125, 128–129, 134,
    137, 139, 140
    defense system of, 52–53
    definition of, 137
arrhythmia, 76, 137
    definition of, 137
arteries, 16, 19, 24–25, 26, 28, 32,
    49–50, 55, 69, 70, 73, 74, 75, 76,
    78, 79, 83, 86, 87, 88, 89–90, 92,
    101, 103, 104, 113, 124, 126,
    127, 128, 137, 138, 139
    definition of, 137
atherosclerosis, 70, 83, 128, 137,
    138, 140
    definition of, 137
atom, 138, 139, 140
    definition of, 137

belladonna, 140
bile (*see* acids, bile)
blood pressure:
    high (*see also* hypertension) 1,
        2, 3, 7, 14, 17, 24–34, 35, 37,
        90, 116, 126, 132, 134, 139
        and connection with fast
            food, 23–34
    optimal, 27, 36, 37
    systolic, 27, 142
blood vessels disease, 137
bran, 114, 137

calcium, 36, 37, 129, 137, 141
cardiovascular disease (CVD), 49,
    55, 73
    definition of, 138
cholesterol:
    definition of, 83–84
    desirable levels of, 85, 87
    HDL, 87–89
    LDL, 86–87
        oxidized, 60, 140
        definition of, 140
coronary artery disease (*see* coro-
    nary heart disease)
coronary heart disease, 78, 138,
    139

DASH sodium trial, 27
diabetes, 16, 39, 138

electron, 49, 51, 52, 138
ellagic acid, 55
endosperm, 114, 138
endothelium, 49–50, 89, 138
enzyme, 52, 54, 56, 130, 138, 140

fat:
    monounsaturated, 74–75, 102,
        140
        definition of, 140
    polyunsaturated, 73, 75, 76,
        102, 140, 141
        definition of, 141
    saturated (*see also* triglycer-
        ides), 28, 69–71, 73, 74, 77,
        79, 84, 89, 90–91, 92, 93,
        101, 102, 141
        and content in meat, 72
        definition of, 141
    trans, 69, 70, 77–81, 84, 90,
        91–92, 93, 142
        definition of, 142
fiber, 8, 16, 32, 109–117, 138
    and link to cholesterol, 112–113
    insoluble, 111, 114, 139
    overview of, 111
    soluble, 111, 112, 114, 115–
        116, 141
fish oil (*see* omega-3 oils)
folic acid, 110, 113, 138
free radicals, 49, 50–52, 54, 60, 75,
    88–90, 128, 137, 138, 140–141
    definition of, 138
    description of, 49–51
fruit:
    fresh versus frozen, 39–40
    importance of in diet, 35

gangrene, 125
    definition of, 139
garlic, 123–135
    and adverse effects from, 133–
        135
    and cholesterol levels, 126–127
    and high blood pressure, 126
    and plaque in arteries, 128
    and platelets, 127
    antioxidant properties of, 124–
        125, 128–129
    as antioxidant, 128–129
    guidelines for cooking with,
        129–130
garlic supplements, 131–132
germ, 114
    definition of, 139
grains, whole, 11, 109–117

heart attack, 2, 8, 14, 15, 16, 17,
    19, 24, 25, 26, 51, 53, 69, 70, 76,
    86, 89, 90, 112, 113, 126, 127,
    139, 141
homocysteine, 113,
    definition of, 139
    description of, 113
hormone, 68, 83, 138
    definition of, 139
hydrocarbons, 104
hydrogenation, 77, 78, 139
    definition of, 139
hypertension (*see also* blood
    pressure, high), 16, 24–28, 37,
    139
    definition of, 139

iron, 73

legumes, 109–117
lipoproteins, 86, 87, 90, 103, 139
    high density, 86, 87
        definition of, 139
lycopene, 53, 60–65, 139
    absorption of, 61–63
    definition of, 60, 139

magnesium, 36–37, 110, 114, 129, 140
    definition of, 140
manganese, 110
Mediterranean diet:
    definition of, 4, 140
    pillars of, 11
metabolism, 50, 140
    definition of, 140
microbe, 29, 140
    definition of, 140
molecule, 4, 37, 49, 50, 51, 77, 89, 139, 140, 141, 142
    definition of, 140
Multiple Risk Factor Intervention Trial, 85

nightshade, 59, 140
    definition of, 140

oil:
    hydrogenated, 77–78, 80, 81, 91, 92, 93, 139
        definition of, 139
    olive, 97–107
        antioxidant properties of, 99, 101, 105, 114
        advantages of frying with, 106
        fat composition of, 101–102
        minor components of, 102, 140
        purchase guidelines for, 105
omega-3 oils, 76–77, 93, 140
    definition of, 140
organic, definition of, 140
oxidants, definition of, 140
oxidation, 49, 50, 51, 60, 61, 75, 88, 89–90, 100, 102, 103, 104, 128, 137, 140
    definition of, 140

pedometer, 21, 141
phosphorous, 110
phytochemical, 53, 54, 141
    definition of, 141
phytochemicals: carotenoids, 55
phytochemicals: flavenoids, 55
placebo, 113, 141
    definition of, 141
plaque, 25, 38, 50, 51, 79, 86, 89, 126, 128, 137, 141, 142
    definition of, 141
platelets, 16, 54, 76, 89, 127–128, 141, 142
    definition of, 141
polyphenols (*see also* antioxidants), 104
potassium, 33, 35, 36, 110, 114, 129, 141

Researchers for the Heart Outcomes Prevention Evaluation Study, 103

selenium, 129
siesta, 6–8, 141
    definition of, 141

sodium:
    and processed foods, 29–34
    steps to lower intake of, 41–43
stroke, 2, 25, 26, 36, 53, 76, 89,
    113, 126, 127, 134, 139, 141
    definition of, 141
    hemorrhagic, 25
        definition of, 139

thrombosis, definition of, 142
thromboxane, definition of, 142
thrombus, 127, 142
    definition of, 142
tomatoes, and heart health *(see also*
    lycopene), 59–65
triglycerides, 1–3, 7, 14, 16, 76, 88,
    124, 127, 133, 138, 139, 140,
    141, 142
    definition of, 2, 142

vegetables:
    fresh versus frozen, 39–40
    importance of in diet, 35
vitamin A, 68, 129
vitamin B1, 129
vitamin B12, 68, 113
vitamin B6, 113
vitamin C, 53, 54, 55, 129
vitamin D, 68, 83
vitamin E, 53, 55, 68, 102–103,
    114, 133
vitamin K, 68
vitamin, multi-, 103
vitamins, definition of, 142

zinc, 73, 110, 139